USEFUL
ADMONITIONS
✛ ## TO THE ✛
CHRISTIAN
NURSE

*A Pragmatic, Theological,
and Empirical Equipoise*

LAWRENCE ONWUEGBUCHUNAM,
Ph.D., RN.

◆ FriesenPress

Suite 300 - 990 Fort St
Victoria, BC, V8V 3K2
Canada

www.friesenpress.com

ISBN
978-1-03-910877-6 (Hardcover)
978-1-03-910876-9 (Paperback)
978-1-03-910878-3 (eBook)

1. RELIGION, CHRISTIAN LIFE, CALLING & VOCATION

Distributed to the trade by The Ingram Book Company

Table of Contents

CHAPTER 1: Historical Perspective of Nursing as a Caring Profession

Nurses dispense comfort, compassion and caring
without even a prescription
—Val Saintsbury

NURSING PRACTICE EMERGED in the context of addressing the needs of the people, with the primary motive of making people feel better to respond to their activities of daily living and function at their optimal level. Nursing practice is not static, but it evolves as the values, beliefs, and knowledge of a society continue to change and improve, especially in the areas of health and illness.

In the early seventeen century, caring for the sick people in an institution such as the hospital was an elusive concept. Nursing and caring for the sick were understood as taking care of an ill person from one's home. The practice of professional nursing can be attributed to Florence Nightingale, who, after receiving training as a nurse, advanced nursing care with the underlying philosophy that it should be anchored in compassion, physical observation, knowledge, and that this should be provided at no cost (Ball, 2013). Florence Nightingale worked at the military hospital during the Crimean War, and during that period, she cared for the sick and the wounded soldiers, reduced overcrowding of the hospital, and reduced the mortality rate of the sick and wounded soldiers (Ball, 2013).

Florence Nightingale advanced nursing practice through her caring process and her writings. She clearly defined the role and scope of nursing, which led to the training of more nurses and the construction of more government hospitals. Through her relentless effort, perseverance, competent care of the sick, and writing, Florence Nightingale established nursing care as a professional practice that is grounded in adequate knowledge. Among the values she demonstrated in her nursing practice and envisioned for the future of nursing were nursing as a vocation (calling), nursing as an art and science, the conviction that people can live optimally through nursing, that nursing requires specific knowledge, and that nursing is distinct from medicine (Ball, 2013). In the following pages, Florence Nightingale's values regarding what nursing is and should become will be explored through the lens of Christian worldview.

Nursing as a Calling and Vocation

Historically, nursing has been perceived as a calling, a vocation anchored in care and service, with a subterranean religious significance (Kerr & MacPhail, 1991). Nursing was positioned as a vocation of care and service, and practising nurses of the early twentieth century did not look forward to much reimbursement and worldly remuneration for their duties (O'Brien, 2011). Rather, nurses perceived caregiving as a calling and a vocation commissioned by God, to whom alone honour and thanksgiving belonged for the care they provided (O'Brien, 2011). The idea of nursing as a vocation of caring and service is well documented in literature (Bradshaw, 2002, Kerr & MacPhail, 1991; O'Brien, 2011). This idea of nursing as a vocation also has both champions and detractors. The champions or the proponents of nursing as a vocation, including Florence Nightingale, believe that nursing is more than a mere choice of career and that nursing has a spiritual component, a destiny that was ordained by God, and a commitment to care and service. Detractors of this idea argue that nursing is merely a career choice that one makes, which has no spiritual or religious significance.

Currently, nursing is perceived as a profession that has no religious significance but is still grounded in care and service (Kerr & MacPhail, 1991). Nursing practice in Canada, for example, is perceived as a practised discipline and political act anchored in care and service (CNA, 2002). Nursing in recent times is perceived as a duty to care for the sick, a profession rather than an altruistic calling. The fact is that nursing can be both a calling as well as a career choice for the Christian nurse. The concepts of nursing as a calling and nursing as a career choice are not mutually exclusive because caring is the underlying altruistic essence or the foundation of nursing practice, and as such, caring can transform the choice of working in the nursing profession into a call to care. It can also change a call to care into a choice of a profession (Carter, 2014). Therefore, for the Christian nurse, it is a statement of fact that nursing professional practice could provide ample opportunity for the actualization, fulfillment, and attainment of the call or the vocation to care for others.

The Idea of Nursing as a Calling and Vocation from Christian Worldview

Christians locate the meaning of vocation within the context of God's calling in life, which suggests that our lives on earth have both meaning and purpose, which is not distant and distinct from reflecting the image of God in whatever occupation we have. Christians believe that God's calling in life implied that they reflect the practices of Jesus, evident in the scriptures, in their personal lives. In other words, the fundamental principles that will determine Christian nurses' actions are anchored in asking the following three foundational questions: what is the best practice or what does the guidelines for nursing practice say? What does the policy and procedure where I work say about a particular action? And what would Jesus do in this particular situation?

The answers to these fundamental questions are significant, since they will serve as the underlying factors that inform and influence the Christian nurse's decision-making process and nursing action. It is important that the Christian nurse cherish and adhere to the guidelines for nursing professional practice while following the policy and protocol in the workplace. These policies, protocols, and professional responsibilities are primarily in place to ensure a safe and competent nursing practice. While the guidelines for nursing practice are essential, they are not impeccable or perfect. They guarantee basic, or rather, above-average nursing practice, and they do not necessarily guarantee nursing practice perfection.

Through my extensive experience and knowledge of nursing practice, especially in the context of frontline nursing care, I have come to see and understand that there is a significant difference between a care that is anchored in simply following the protocols in place because the nurse doesn't want to get into trouble, and a care that involved the total giving of self of the nurse, with the knowledge and the understanding that the nurse is the person at the service of patients' needs. Some of us can easily name many nurses who show up to work simply because they need to make an honest living. The idea of just making an honest living is not to be perceived as something evil, because it isn't. Some of us can also easily name nurses who come to work and involve the totality of who they are and what they believe in caring for their patients, and are happy to serve the needs of the patients. The difference in care provided between these categories of nurses is simply clear. What then is the meaning and the context of caring in nursing?

In an effort to create a clear picture of what nurses do in the context of their caring for patients, Roach (2002) identified the six C's of caring as follows: compassion, competence, confidence, conscience, commitment, and comportment. These essential components of caring in nursing have underlying spiritual and theological significance.

Compassion is an effort by the nurse to genuinely experience what the patient is experiencing (Roach, 2002). In this context, the meaning of compassion is very close to empathy. I love to describe empathy in the context of role-playing. Here, nurses attempt to step out of their roles and put themselves in the shoes of the patients, trying to have a better understanding of what the patient is going through. This approach could enable the nurse to make the necessary adjustment to experience the pain, the fears, and the expectation of patients and their families, in order to create an intervention that is patient- and family-centred, as well as appropriate and effective.

We have instances in the Bible where Jesus was filled with compassion for the people and where Jesus applied empathy while relating with the people, and he was moved to take actions to alleviate their needs, pain and suffering. In the gospel of Luke, Jesus saw a dead man who was a widow's only child, and the widow was in pain due to the death of her only son. Jesus was moved with compassion, and then he told the woman not to weep. Looking at the dead son, Jesus said, "Young man I say unto to thee arise" (Luke 7:14). Also, in the gospel of Matthew, Jesus was moved with compassion for the multitude of very hungry people who came to listen to His teaching for an extensive period of time. This compassion moved Jesus to action, to perform a miracle and feed the multitude, and they ate to their satisfaction.

Competence is an essential aspect of the meaning of caring in nursing practice. Competence is the nurse's ability to possess the knowledge of the illness the patient is experiencing to effectively intervene with treatment. For nurses to demonstrate competent care, they must be equipped with the right knowledge about patients' conditions. They must also be experts in assessing the physical, spiritual, and psychological needs of patients, with the ability to provide treatments and explore resources that are relevant to patients' recovery in holistic context. Christian nurses should be able to re-evaluate the care they provide to patients to ensure that the care is both effective and specific to each patient's needs. The Christian nurse should do everything necessary to practise competently, in line with the Letter of St. Paul to Timothy, where Paul advised Timothy to strive to be the best worker who is rightly approved and who does not need to be ashamed due to impediments or lacks (2 Timothy 2:15).

Confidence, another aspect of caring in nursing, is an important quality for a nurse to acquire. Christian nurses should be able to demonstrate with confidence that they have the right knowledge and the experience to care for patients. The confidence to demonstrate the possession of appropriate knowledge about patients' conditions could facilitate trust by patients and their families. A nurse who practises with confidence is sharply in contrast with a nurse who practises with pride and arrogance. Confidence here is grounded in the nurse's cognitive humility and assertiveness. Confidence, when rightly applied in the clinical settings, could facilitate the development of a trusting relationship between the patient and the nurse. The Christian nurse should practise with confidence that is grounded in faith and in God, with the knowledge that God commanded us to "be strong and courageous. Do not be afraid; do not be discouraged, for the Lord will go with you wherever you go" (Joshua 1:9). The Psalmist exclaimed: "even when I walk in the valley of shadow of death, no evil will I fear, for you are with me; your rod and your staff, they comfort me." (Psalm 27:3). Indeed, "those who put their hope in the Lord will renew their strength. They will soar on wings like eagles; they will run and not grow weary; they will walk and not faint." (Isaiah 40:31). Confidence that is anchored in God, humility, and knowledge, should resonate with every Christian nurse.

Conscience is an aspect of nursing care that deals with the rational process that evokes emotional and cognitive judgment based on one's moral values and moral philosophy. For the Christian nurse, conscience is part of our moral compass. Our values and morals inform and influence our decisions and actions. The nurse's conscience should inform them about the right action to take in any clinical situation, while making sure that patients' rights are not violated. It should guide the nurse to provide patients with the right information, without giving them false hope, and without withholding any information that would enable patients to make informed decision (Roach, 2002). While caring for patients, Christian nurses should demonstrate emotional and cognitive knowledge through the lens of moral values enshrined in their conscience.

Commitment, as an attribute of nursing care, is the nurse's obligation and engagement with the care and the needs of the patients. Christian nurses should understand that they have the obligation to fully immerse themselves in the care of the patients. In other words, give the patient a sense of commitment and solidarity; let them know that both of you are in this journey of recovery together. Love is central to making commitments. This love should be grounded in the principle of "Golden Rule." The Christian nurse should always remember the word of Jesus to "do unto others as you would want them to do to you" (Luke 6:31). This biblical passage should be a conscious reminder for the Christian nurse to stay solidly grounded in the commitment to the care of patients.

Comportment, as an attribute of caring in nursing, is essential. The Christian nurse should comport themselves in a professional manner and in accordance with the ethical and moral principles that inform nursing practice. The nurses' appearance and language while caring for patients should be grounded in professionalism, knowledge, and constructive emotion. The nurse should appear neatly and seriously. They should maintain an appearance that aligns with decency and business, which could translate to being perceived as someone who is serous by the patient and their families. The Christian nurse should be consciously aware of the need to conduct themselves in a manner that is worthy of the message of Christ, as evident in the letter of St. Paul to the Philippians (Philippians 1:27).

It is a privilege for a Christian to be a nurse. This privilege also demands a commitment and a responsibility to offer one's whole self to the care of patients, to extend the mission of Christ to the sick and the broken-hearted, and to heal the wounded. If Christian nurses truly understand the idea that their nursing profession is a vocation given to them by God—who is their source of inspiration to be a nurse in the first place, who provided them with the resources they needed on their journey toward becoming nurses, and who supported them through the rigorous nursing training—it could help them to see, and easily understand, the purpose that God has for them in their nursing profession.

Evident in the Bible is the fact that sometimes, God's inspirations and callings for us as Christians are not always clear. Sometimes, God's calling comes with challenges and uncomfortable demands. In the first book of Samuel, Chapter 3, when God called Samuel, Samuel misunderstood the voice of God and the inspiration from God. But with the support of Eli, Samuel later understood and recognized the voice of God, and he responded to his calling. There are several instances in the Bible where people didn't initially recognize the call of God and the inspiration from God in their lives, and where people judged themselves as incapable of responding to God's calling due to their perceived impediments and limitations. Later, with the grace and support of God, they were able to recognize and discern God's will for them, and responded to the calling of God

Every Christian nurse has their own experience, narrative, and story of the inspiration from God to be a nurse, although those stories may have similarities and differences from one person to the other. Some of us were more aware of our strengths and desires to care for the people in the context of nursing. Some of us may have had the underlying desire to care for people but were not sure whether we had what it takes, both intellectually and otherwise, to commit to a nursing program and nursing preparations, due to our perceived self-impediments or lacks. It is correct to say that even though God has a purpose and a plan for our lives as Christians, God also respects our choices and our freedom to choose. But, in most cases, God has a way of keeping the calling or the vocation He has for us to a particular career alive in our minds, despite our doubts about our abilities. God also moves in mysterious ways, and as such, could provide people and resources on our ways, to continue to inflame or keep the desires within us alive. Often, "God chose the foolish in the world to shame the wise; God chose the weak to shame the strong (1 Corinthians 1:27).

The calling from God is not always clear and linear. Sometimes, we may be heading in one direction due to our internal desires or the stage we are in our lives, whereas God may have different plans for our lives. Using the story of my life as an example, most of my childhood life and significant adult life, I knew that I loved to care for people, I knew that caring and service were some of my strengths, and I spent significant amount of time in post-secondary education in preparation to become a pastor. As I continue to grow and to know myself, and after years of scrupulous examinations and rigorous discernment, I left the seminary training, happily married, had children, and channelled my desire to care and serve through nursing. I am very happy as a person, and I am very fulfilled in my nursing profession. Sometimes, some of us may go through different routes before we find our calling in life. It is not a waste of time, and if we trust in the providence of God, we will understand that God used those different experiences to prepare us for what and where He knows we will be happy and fulfilled. Every experience we may go through in life is preparing us for the vocation and the plan of God in our lives, which is often better and greater.

So, what then? How should we, as Christians, respond to our vocation and choice of nursing as a profession? From a Christian worldview and perspective, a vocation or calling from God is simply an opportunity for the ministry, to represent and reflect the life of Christ in everything we do, including our job. For Christian nurses, therefore, nursing becomes an opportunity to touch the lives of the people they meet, to care for the sick, to contribute to healing the broken-hearted, to bandage the wounded, to feed the hungry, to give water to the thirsty, to help the weary find rest, to calm the anxious, and to open the door to the homeless.

For a Christian nurse to faithfully respond to nursing vocation from a Christian perspective, the nurse should first make room in their heart. Nursing profession is anchored in the acts of hospitality, and hospitality as a way of life is both fundamental and foundational to the meaning and identity of Christians (Pohl, 1999). By making room in their hearts to care for the sick, the weary, the anxious and the broken-hearted, to mention but a few, Christian nurses are allowing and giving God permission to use them as instruments to extend His ministry to the people they meet and to reflect His presence both in words and in actions to the world.

For the Christian nurse, the call to the profession of nursing is a call to a life of hospitality and caring. In the Old Testament tradition, hospitality was perceived and under-stood as the foundation of moral structure, which included welcoming strangers, the sick, and the hungry, to mention but a few. Hospitality is also central in the New Testament tradition (Pohl, 1999). Nursing hospitality therefore begins with a loving and generous predisposition of the heart of the nurse. This internal predisposition should then translate to outward manifestation through the words and the actions of the Christian nurse to competent nursing practice, grounded in knowledge and regulated emotion.

In order for Christian nurses to competently respond to the nursing vocation, they need a total surrender to God, and a total reliance on the grace of God, to touch the lives of the people that they meet at work. The nurse should understand that their nursing practice, which is their source of livelihood and sustenance, is also an opportunity to make a difference in the lives of the people, in line with their call to Christian life in the first place.

Total dependence on the will and the grace of God means that the Christian nurse should make prayer a habit and a second nature. Christian nurses should begin and end their work with prayer. While at work, especially but not exclusively before performing any difficult task or meeting a difficult patient, the nurse should present those moments to God in prayer, asking for the grace to respond competently to the work at hand and to allow people to meet Christ through their presence.

The Christian nurse should also make reflection and meditation essential components of their nursing practice. At the end of each workday, Christian nurses should devote a significant time in reflecting on the actions they took while at work, ensuring that they aligned with the policy and protocols in the workplace and that they bore the image of Christ at work. This reflective practice is an opportunity for the nurse to ask fundamental questions, such as, "What did I learn from a particular experience with a patient?" and "What will I do differently in the future?"

Reflective practice helps the Christian nurse continue to grow in knowledge and in practice in the context of continuing nursing competence. It helps the Christian nurse to identify personal and professional strengths and weaknesses, and it helps nurses to be consciously aware of their educational needs and find areas to improve.

But humility is necessarily important in productive reflective practice. Humility is a necessary tool for the Christian nurse to identify weaknesses and areas to improve. Humility is the ability to have an honest and modest look at one's practice for a potential revelation of strengths and weaknesses. A humble Christian nurse, who is open and receptive to constructive criticisms, is on the path to great achievements.

CHAPTER 2: The Spiritual Component of Nursing

We are not human beings having spiritual experience. We are spiritual beings having human experience.
—Pierre Teilhard de Chardin.

SPIRITUALITY HAS BEEN explained as the individual's deep sense of connection, through which one finds meaning and purpose in life and gains a sense of belonging and acceptance (Dein, Cook, Powell & Eagger, 2010). There is lack of clarity and specificity around the meaning and the context of spirituality in professional nursing. The empirical content of nursing appears to be getting more attention and more emphasis due to its scientific nature. Spirituality, on the other hand, is rarely discussed in nursing school or professional nursing, even though spirituality is an essential component of holistic nursing practice (Petterson, 1998).

The idea of holistic nursing assessment and intervention as the content and the context of understanding competent nursing is getting popular among clinicians and nursing scholars. For nurses, spiritual assessment is a compulsory component of effective nursing assessment that covers the holistic health and well-being of patients. For health care professionals, including nurses, to be competent in the assessment and intervention of patients' spiritual needs, they need to understand each patient's cultural context and the context of their own practice before making any clinical judgment (Fallot, 2001).

From an historical perspective, Florence Nightingale, the founder of nursing, envisioned nursing as a vocation from God, which also has a spiritual component. I argue that nursing practice has a spiritual component, since caring, service, and hospitality, to mention but a few, which are fundamental to nursing practice, are also foundational to spiritual and religious practice. I contend that human beings are composed beings by nature. Much of the theological and philosophical cannons asserts that humans are composed of body and soul, the material and the spiritual (immaterial). Following Aristotle's philosophy, Thomas Aquinas argued that body (matter) and soul (form), though distinct, are inseparable, and as such, one cannot see a body without a soul or a soul without a body (Stumpf, 2008). Therefore, following this line of thought, one can argue that spirituality is an essential component of human beings and that the search for meaning and purpose is embedded in the very nature of humans. Nurses' patients have both physical and spiritual needs. Since patients that nurses work with have a spiritual component and spiritual needs, spirituality is an indispensable component of holistic and competent nursing practice.

However, it is a statement of fact, grounded in empirical evidence, that some nurses do not include spiritual assessments in their patients' assessments and interventions (Rousseau, 2000). There is also a fundamental lack of spiritual assessment and a lack of emphasis on the importance of spirituality in nursing academic curriculum. The nurses' inability to include spiritual assessments in their nursing practice can be attributed to their lack of knowledge or incompetence in spiritual assessment. It could also be due to fear of being judged or reprimanded, as we have seen cases where nurses were punished for engaging in prayer with their patients. Whatever the reason may be, it does not justify the apparent lack or inadequacy of the spiritual assessment and spiritual intervention seen in nursing practice. This fundamental lack of competent spiritual assessment and intervention impedes the realization or actualization of a holistic nursing practice.

The forms of spirituality and spiritual care in nursing practice can vary from one patient to another, and from one designated nursing care or hospital facility to others, as long as it fits the spiritual needs of the patients in the context of patient-centred care. Nurses and other health care professionals can incorporate spiritual assessment as their routine practice, develop group therapeutic treatment that addresses spiritual issues, incorporate spirituality in psychotherapy, and provide their patients with opportunities for community spiritual supports (Fallot, 2001).

It is even more pertinent that Christian nurses assess and address their clients' spiritual needs. The Christian nurse should develop listening ears to be able to accurately assess clients' concern around meaning and purpose in life. Depending on where clients are in their recovery journey and their readiness/willingness to explore questions around their spirituality, the Christian nurse should perceive spiritual assessment as a vital component of competent nursing practice. During the nurses' therapeutic communication and assessment of the patients' needs, the Christian nurse should not shy away from the discussion around the patients' religious or spiritual needs, especially, but not exclusively, when the patient has identified spirituality as a meaningful coping mechanism in their life. To the best of my knowledge of nursing best practices, there is nothing that forbids a nurse from having a healthy discussion with the patient on the topics around spirituality, especially in the context of spiritual assessment.

The Christian nurse should also be extremely cautious not to use nursing professional practice as an avenue for Christian evangelization by preaching to the patient. The Christian nurse should primarily take the role of a listener and stay where their patients are to effectively respond to the patients' needs. The Christian nurse should be very cautious not to tell their clients what they think or what they believe their clients should do while assessing their spiritual needs. A Christian nurse's major task during spiritual assessments should be listening to, and validating, clients' spiritual needs and emotions, exploring and processing those needs with the client, and being ready to make referrals for further spiritual supports and resources available and approved in a designated nursing care facility.

If spirituality and prayer are meaningful to the client, and if the client requests prayer from the nurse, there is nothing wrong in the Christian nurses' assertion and promise to keep their clients in their personal prayers in order to continue to find meaning and purpose in their illness journey and recovery. Also, the Christian nurse should make it a habit to keep their clients in their personal prayer, though they don't necessarily have to tell their clients that they are praying for them. The Christian nurse should understand that praying for the living and the dead is one of the Seven Spiritual Works of Mercy that Christians are called to perform. Whenever a Christian nurse sees a patient struggling with meaning and purpose in life, especially when the patient is confronted with terminal illness, the nurse has a Christian obligation to keep that client in their personal prayers, without telling the patient, regardless of whether the patient has any spiritual or religious belief.

The Christian nurse should also be consciously aware of the fact that faith without good work is dead (James 2:17). In other words, the Christian nurse should strive to live up to what they believe during patient care. It is necessary to go the extra mile while caring for the patient. While caring for the patient, those simple nursing duties such as listening to the patient, medication administration, and feeding the patient, to mention but a few, should be done in an extraordinary way. The Christian nurse should not strive to do extraordinary things while caring for the patient. Rather, they should do their daily nursing duties in extraordinary ways. While going the extra mile in caring for the patient, the Christian nurse should offer those sacrifices silently in prayer to God. By offering those sacrifices to God in prayer, the job that is a means of honest living and decent pay could also be a means for blessings, graces from God, and a way to respond to the call to live a Christian life.

The reality is that the idea of spirituality in nursing is deeply rooted in the notion of holistic nursing care. Spirituality is often understood in the context of meaning, purpose, and values that have outward manifestation and expression in human attributes, such as love, caring, compassion, honesty, and sincerity, to mention but a few.

Spirituality in Christian context suggests a belief in the existence of metaphysical, supernatural, and transcendental reality—God, who is both immanent and transcendent. In the Christian worldview, God's divine transcendence does not mean that God is so far from His people, or that God is so distant from humans that the relationship with God becomes an elusive concept. Rather, it means that God, who is a transcendental and supreme being, is equally involved with His people in a personal and covenantal way.

Spirituality in Christian contexts is anchored in the belief in the existence of an immanent transcendent God who is all-loving, all-powerful, all-knowing, and the source of everything that is good. God is everywhere—in the heaven above, and on the earth below. God does not watch His creatures from a distance; He participates in the world He created. The psalmist beautifully described the nature of the immanent transcendent God in the book of psalms chapter 139: 7-12 as follows:

Where can I go from your spirit? Where can I flee from your presence?

If I go up to heavens, you are there; if I make my bed in depths, you are there.

If I rise on the wings of the dawn, if I settle on the far side of the sea, even there your hand will guide me, your right hand will hold me fast. If I say, "Surely the darkness will hide me, and the light become night around me" even the darkness is not dark to you; the night will shine like the day, for darkness is as light to you.

Therefore, for the Christian nurse, it is necessary to be consciously aware of God's immanent transcendent nature and the fact that God is always close to them, including to the patients entrusted to their care. It is a common belief in the Christian worldview that human beings are created in the image and likeness of God, a statement of faith that is evident in the Bible. Spirituality is the channel through which Christian nurses maintain their relationship with God and connect with God. The Christian nurse should also see the image of the invincible God in the patients they serve.

The role of healthy spirituality in patients' recovery is robustly documented in literature. Ross (1994) under-scored the importance of spirituality in nursing practice and contended that spiritual care is the nurse's responsibility, a responsibility within the nurse's scope of practice, rather than optional or extra work for the nurse. In line with this thought process, Roy (1984) acknowledged that nurses should partici-pate in meeting patients' spiritual needs.

Spirituality is important to most of the patients that nurses work with. In order to explore the right answers, it is neces-sary to ask the right question about why some nurses pay less attention or place less value on the relevancy of spiritual assessments and spiritual interventions in patients' recovery and wellness journey. The logical answer to this fundamental question could be underpinned by the fact that the scientific paradigm is often favoured, worshipped, and adored in nursing practice, with a subterranean suspicion and perception of spirituality as vague and unscientific. It could also be associated with the fact that some nurses are uncomfortable with the notion of incorporating spirituality in their practice due to their lack of competency with the knowledge of spiritual assessment and intervention.

Whatever the reason may be, it does not excuse, exonerate, or justify the fundamental privation or lack of spiritual assessment and the inadequacy of spiritual assessment and intervention in nursing practice. Depriving patients of the necessary spiritual support they need is equivalent to depriving them of access to essential coping skills that are vital to their recovery.

The Christian nurse should perceive the assessment of the patients' spiritual needs as equally important, just as the assessment of patients' physical and psychological needs are in the context of holistic nursing practice. The Christian nurse should ground their spiritual assessment and intervention to meet the needs of patients within the guidelines set by the regulatory bodies, as well as in accordance with the guidelines and protocols in their workplace. The Christian nurse needs to be polite, assertive and, in a non-confrontational manner, advocate for the inclusion of spiritual assessment and spiritual intervention in the facilities where they work, if it is not already incorporated in the patients' care plan.

CHAPTER 3: Workplace Violence in Nursing

Man must evolve for all human conflict a method
which rejects revenge, aggression, and retaliation.
The foundation of such method is love.
—Martin Luther King, Jr.

IT IS A common saying, both in nursing school and in nursing professional practice, that nurses eat their young and, sometimes, eat each other. I remember the last theory course I took while in nursing school, which goes with the final year clinical practical course called "Issues in Nursing Professional Practice." During this course, the clear picture of different ways aggression and hostility could manifest in nursing was discussed, and to prepare us both mentally and emotionally about this potential abuse, emphasis was particularly placed on the fact that some nurses do eat their young.

The existence of hostility and aggression in nursing cannot be denied, and it is well documented in nursing literature. It is a fact that a lot of nurses care for the patients and support their colleagues. It is also evident that in some workplaces, some nurses eat their young and one another. The hostility in nursing could come from a fellow nurse who is on the same level with you. It could also come from the nurse who is in management or leadership role and is above you. Wherever the source of hostility and aggression is, it should not be tolerated or condoned.

There is a variety of ways that nurses show hostility and aggression to one another, such as bullying, verbal abuse, harassment, aggression (both active and passive), anger, withholding important information, name calling, backstabbing, destructive criticisms, gossip, creating unfair patient assignment, fault-finding, using put-downs, refusing to help a struggling nurse, isolation, and exclusion, to mention but a few (Bartholomew, 2006).

How can a Christian nurse thrive and excel in this kind of workplace environment? What options does a Christian nurse have in a nursing hostile environment? The least a Christian nurse should do is make sure that they are not part of the perpetrators of hostility and aggression in the workplace, either directly or indirectly. Most of us have in one way or another experienced some form of hostility and aggression in the workplace at some point. Even if you have not experienced it directly yourself, you may have seen it or know somebody who has experienced it. Evidently, it will be incredibly naïve to think or to believe that the above-mentioned different ways of hostility and aggression cannot be experienced in nursing professional practice.

Although violence in nursing can take various forms, including physical violence, Houston (2006) noted that physical violence in nursing does not occur as frequently as non-physical attacks. There are other ways nurses experience violence in the workplace, ranging from patients to the nurses, from doctors to nurses, and from nurse to nurse, to mention but a few. The focus here is on violence and aggression from nurse to nurse.

Houston (2006) identified seven categories of violence in nursing, as follows: internal violence, client-initiated violence, organizational violence, external violence, third-party violence, nursing work violence, and nurse-initiated violence. The reality is that violence of any category to nurses, especially nurse-to-nurse violence, often negatively impacts the nurse who is the victim of abuse, physically, socially, mentally, and otherwise.

An example of extreme case of negative impact of nurse-to-nurse violence was a situation where the perpetrator of the violence was a senior nurse, and the victim was a younger nurse. The abuse triggered suicidal ideas for the nurse who was the receiver of the abuse (Houston, 2006). The impact of workplace violence on the mind and the mental health of the nurse who is the victim of the abuse could translate to serious mental illness, such as anxiety, depression, and post-traumatic stress disorder. These mental health issues could also translate to burnout issues.

The reality is that health is understood in a holistic context, and all the human organs are interconnected and interdependent on each other to function well so that the individual could function at the optimal level. In other words, workplace violence has emotional symptoms, such as anger and irritability, on the nurse who is the receiver of the violence. Socially, it could trigger lack of self-confidence, low self-esteem, lack of connectedness with the team, and lack of sense of belonging for the nurse who is the victim of workplace abuse. Physiologically, workplace violence and aggression could lead to cardiac problems and other health problems to the victim.

I counsel the Christian nurse not to operate with the ideology of an eye for an eye and a tooth for a tooth as a response to nursing workplace hostility and aggression. Do not love only the nurse who loves you while hating the nurse who despises you. But rather, "love your enemy and pray for those who persecute you" (Matthew 5:44). In another passage in the Bible, where the pharisees came to test Jesus to find fault with Him, they asked Jesus which was the greatest commandment. Jesus' response was fascinating: "thou shall love the Lord thy God with all your heart, soul and mind, and your neighbour as yourself. For these are the summary of the Law and the Prophets" (Matthew 22: 35-40). Folks, these statements are brilliant. It is crystal clear, therefore, that love is both fundamental and foundational to the meaning, the content, and the context of what it means to be a Christian. It is necessary for the Christian nurse to remember that the first intervention in response to workplace violence in nursing is to show love to the nurse who is the perpetrator of violence, and as well, to keep that nurse in prayer. As Christians, prayer is the greatest weapon we have, and it is through prayer that we communicate to God, whom we believe is greater than any problem we may have in life. So, prayer is the highest weapon that the Christian nurse has.

Remember that there is a reason why God tells us to love everyone, including the people who persecute us. With love, we can conquer hate. Jesus himself has shown us what it means to love someone. The death on the cross for us sinners is a constant reminder of the need to love everyone, both champions and detractors. To love genuinely demands some degree of sacrifice and pain bearing. The example that Jesus demonstrated on the cross is agape love, which is an unconditional love of the other. It is the same love that we are called as Christians to show to everyone. As human beings, it is extremely difficult to love the person who despises us and who causes us a lot of pain. It is necessary that I stress this obvious fact. But when we bear grudges as Christians, we live in bondage. We run the risks of losing the forgiveness of God, as is evident in the Lord's prayer: "Forgive us our sins as we forgive those who sinned against us" (Lk. 11:4). It is a conditional prayer. It simply implies that the extent we forgive those who sinned against us is the extent we want God to forgive us our sins. And if we fail to forgive others, we will be living in bondage of sins, and our sins will not be forgiven. We are giving our antagonists power over us. We are losing, and they are winning.

The second response to hostility and aggression in the workplace is for the Christian nurse to engage in assertive communication with the nurse who is the source of violence or hostility. Assertive communication skills enable the Christian nurse to express both the positive and the negative ideas and feelings that they experienced in an open, honest, and non-confrontational way. Assertive communication facilitates constructive and thoughtful conversation and deliberation to find a satisfying solution to conflicts. Through assertive communication skills, the Christian nurse should address the hostile and aggressive behaviour of a colleague that negatively impacts them, express how they feel about the particular bullying behaviour, and strategically communicate their expectations in the future to avoid the reoccurrence of the same behaviour.

The Christian nurse should avoid using unhealthy communication styles, such as passive aggressive communication. Passive aggressive communication is where the Christian nurse develops a pattern of suppressing their feelings and emotions and fails to express their feeling and assert their opinions. Then, when it reaches their high tolerance threshold, they explode and burst, usually out of proportion, intensity, and context, causing a scandal and an unprofessional behaviour in the workplace.

The Christian nurse should be consciously aware of the fact that appropriate timing and the manner of approach are necessary and could translate to effective and successful communication outcome. It is important that the Christian nurse approach a colleague who is the perpetrator of the abuse in the workplace at the right time, when the atmosphere is conducive for communication, especially, when both parties' adrenaline is low or settled. It is equally important for the Christian nurse to take a non-confrontational stance during this process and use the assertive communication skills to make needs known.

If the behaviour of abuse or hostility persists after engaging in assertive communication with the perpetrator of abuse, the Christian nurse should tap into the resources available in the workplace, such as speaking with the manager, the human resources, or the conflict liaison person for support and further intervention. It may be necessary to report the staff to the nursing licensing body only as a last resort. During the whole process, the Christian nurse has the obligation to place everything in the hands of God through prayer and rely on God to fight the battle for them, while simultaneously taking the necessary steps to address the problem, for God sometimes uses human instruments to fight the battle for us.

Sometimes, in very rare instances, the problem could persist, and the hostility and abuse could continue to happen even after the Christian nurse has done all the right things and had followed the necessary steps to resolve the workplace violence. This is where I think that God is testing your Christian faith, and it is the time to trust in divine providence. If Christian nurses fully trust in God's time and believe that whatever God allows them to experience may be in preparation for something potentially greater in the future and that may be an opportunity to step them up for success or progress, then they will be at peace. If the opposite is the case, then they will be going through a lot of emotional difficulty and anxiety. The reality is, in life, sometimes, we have to leave where we are to get to where God wants us to be. It always pays to trust in God while taking the right and the necessary steps when you encounter bullying and hostility of any kind in the workplace.

It is important that the Christian nurse does not fall into the trap of hypersensitivity and hypervigilance in the context of being paranoid and suspicious of other nurses. Hypersensitivity and hypervigilance are the enhanced state of mind where the Christian nurse has exaggerated behaviour and vigilance in a suspicious manner, which translate to perpetual scanning of the workplace environment, looking for, interpreting wrongly, and wrongly perceiving the behaviours of other nurses as being abusive, where there is no evidence or fact that supports such claims. Lastly, it is important for the Christian nurse to take good care of their mental health and understand the reality that sometimes, when a person is sick, that sickness could negatively impact the neurotransmitters in the brain, leading to a mental health crisis known as psychosis, which is loosely explained as a break from reality. This condition could negatively impact the nurse's Christian belief and could lead to what mental health care professionals often refer to as delusions of religious type. If the Christian nurse experiences this type of mental health crisis, spirituality and pharmacologic intervention, in a complementary sense, should be perceived as both necessary and compulsory aspects of treatment, especially, but not exclusively, when there are psychotic symptoms (hallucination and delusion) involved.

Sometimes, in coping with the impact of workplace violence and aggression, the Christian nurse who is the victim of the abuse may need to seek professional help, such as counselling, especially when the trauma from the abuse appears to be negatively impacting the nurse's level of functioning. There is nothing wrong about the Christian nurse to seeking professional help. It does not suggest weakness; rather, it is an important self-care strategy or coping mechanism.

I admonish the Christian nurse to remember that the same Bible that said, "a thousand may fall at your side, ten thousand at your right hand, but it will not come near you" (Psalm 91: 7), also said that "the righteous person may have a lot of troubles, but the Lord will deliver him from them all" (Psalm 34:19). Sure, obstacles, both internal and external, could befall the Christian nurse from anywhere, including the work settings. If Christian nurses persevere in faith and continue to trust and love God, they will eventually see that "for those who love God, all things work together for good" (Romans 8:28). Trusting in God, who is all-loving, all-powerful, and all-knowing, while taking the necessary steps within our human power to end the aggression and violence in the workplace, is just the right thing to do for the Christian nurse.

CHAPTER 4: Whistleblowing and Reporting Misconducts in Nursing Practice

The purpose of whistleblowing is to expose secret and wrongful acts by those in power in order to enable reform.
—Glen Greenwald

THE CONCEPT OF whistleblowing has been in existence in nursing from time immemorial. Whistleblowing is the process of exposing illegal or unlawful acts by creating public awareness about the wrongdoing, including negligence (Kao, 2001). The Canadian Nurses Association (1999) explained whistleblowers as those "who expose negligence, abuses or dangers, such as professional misconduct or incompetence, which exist in organization which they work… It should be considered a last step when all else has failed" (p.1). Sometimes, the consequences the whistleblower go through can be unpleasant and life changing (Ashurst, 2009). Whistleblowing in nursing practice can be explained as the disclosure of unsafe nursing practice or unsafe care provided by health care professionals, including health care institutions to the public. The unpleasant experiences that nurses go through in the process of reporting unprofessional or unsafe nursing or health care practices can be demoralizing and discouraging to nurses who have the intention to do the right thing but are afraid of the potential fallouts or consequences of whistleblowing.

The nurses' actions and decisions in their workplace directly impact the lives of patients, especially, but not exclusively, due to the fact that nurses have access to different kinds of medications in the process of doing their job (Keatings &Smith, 2000). In some states and provinces, such as Alberta and New Brunswick in Canada, it is both the ethical and legal duty of the nurse to report a colleague who has acted in an unprofessional manner, who lacks the skills and the knowledge needed for competent nursing, and whose behaviour, such as addiction to drug and alcohol, or whose mental and physical illness, compromise patients' safety (Keatings & Smith, 200). In those places for example, whistleblowing is not only an ethical responsibility, but a professional responsibility as well, especially when the internal resources have been explored and failed.

Indeed, "the ethical and legal aspects of professional competence, misconduct and malpractice are interrelated. Two means by which the skill and conduct of nurses are gauged are civil law and complaints procedure related to the disciplinary powers of nursing regulatory bodies" (Keatings & Smith,

2000, p. 155). The nurse's actions can negatively affect the lives of the citizens. Nurses have been given right and power to perform a vital duty by the public, and the public in return demands a high level of ethical and competent care from the nurse. The nursing regulatory bodies, especially the Canadian Nurses Association, demands that nurses protect the quality of nursing care and take both preventative and corrective actions to protect patients from unsafe nursing practice, and one of the ways to realize that is through whistleblowing and ongoing effort by the nurse to maintain competence in practice (Keating & Smith, 2000).

The information reported through whistleblowing is often investigated. The investigation process takes different stages, including interviewing the person who witnessed the nurse's action and the victim of the nurse's unsafe or unprofessional practice. The emotions that flow from this investigative process can include relief for the nurse whistleblower, who has done the right thing, as well as the fear of the consequences and unpleasant experiences that come with whistleblowing. Practically speaking, whistleblowing often comes with mixed emotions. Evident in nursing literature and the media are instances where whistleblowing in nursing practice led to improved nursing practice, as well as cases where the nurse who blew the whistle got punished through many other avenues, including job termination, at the extreme.

It is not a guarantee that nurses who blow the whistle are always protected from all kinds of consequences, including alienation from fellow nursing colleagues, bullying, and other obstacles, both internal and external. Sometimes, it may look like nurses who blow the whistle have so much to lose and very little to gain from the process. But the public has a lot to lose if the nurse is not speaking up against unsafe practices in health care (Miller, 2013).

Houston (2006) identified two different types of whistle-blowing: internal whistleblowing and external whistleblowing. Internal whistleblowing is usually a way of creating an aware-ness of an issue to the leadership or the management team within the organization, with the hope that the issue brought forward will be addressed and, hopefully, resolved. External whistleblowing, on the other hand, is simply creating an awareness of a problem outside of the organization, especially, but not exclusively, through the media (Houston, 2006).

The reality of ethical and moral misconduct in businesses, organizations, leadership, and management positions, are both obvious and odious, and they are well documented in scholarly literature. Despite the legislative measures put in place to control ethical and moral issues, including abuse and negligence, the presence of these anomalies cannot be denied.

Indeed, moral courage is an indispensable component of whistleblowing. Knowing the right thing to do, especially when there is an ethical misconduct or when patients' safety is compromised, does not necessarily guarantee or translate to doing the right thing, given that the risks that accompany whistleblowing are often significant.

An extensive review of literature revealed several instances of whistleblowing in nursing practice about issues such as unsafe nursing practice, inadequate nursing staffing, elderly abuse, stealing of patients' narcotics, and fraud, to mention but a few. Houston (2006) noted an instance where nurses were encouraged and advised to participate in falsifying and changing medical records, as well as participate in a cover-up following unjust employment practices.

A prominent case that described the negative impact of whistleblowing in nursing was that of Mary Hochman, who committed suicide in 2002 instead of facing the anger of her supervisor after she reported horrible care, including negligence and the abuse of patients in a care home (Houston, 2006). Indeed, it is important to underscore that external whistleblowing should never be used as a first line of intervention in addressing unethical behaviour or unsafe nursing practice, but it should be used after all other necessary and appropriately established internal protocols and avenues for addressing problems have been used and have failed.

Nurses have an ethical and professional responsibility to speak up when or where there is any abusive, unsafe, and unethical behaviour in nursing practice. The nurse who believes that certain procedures at a workplace prevent them from doing what they know and believe is the right thing could experience moral distress. The moral distress could stem from the fact that nurses have professional obligations to the patients as well as to the employer. This moral distress could lead the nurse to blow the whistle.

The constructive impacts of whistleblowing could lead to changes and innovations that are needed to control and eliminate unsafe practices, ethical and moral misconduct, and negligence. Eradicating these obstacles could translate to improved quality of nursing care for patients. The perils of whistleblowing can also be costly. In extreme cases, as mentioned earlier, it could lead to a job termination of the nurse who blew the whistle, and it could cause emotional and psychological chaos that could trigger the nurse who blew the whistle to experience suicidal ideas and suicide attempts.

What then will a Christian nurse do in difficult and challenging situations of whistleblowing? What option or obligation does a Christian nurse have? Evident in the gospel is the story of the good Samaritan who proved to be a good neighbour to his fellow citizen, to whom the armed robbers showed tremendous violence and aggression and left to the point of death. The good Samaritan went out of his way to care for this stranger in need and took care of him, to the point that Jesus advised the man who asked, "who and how should one be a good neighbour?" to go and do just as the good Samaritan did. That action of the good Samaritan is what I simply describe as practical Christianity, which is the alignment of faith in action. Christian nurses should act like the good Samaritan in rendering care to their patients. Christian nurses therefore have to align their faith in their nursing practice and aim to put themselves in the shoes of the victim who was impacted by the nurse's unsafe practice, especially in following the complaint process established by the regulatory bodies. The Christian nurse should also put themselves in the shoes of the nurse they are reporting. Nurses should ensure that their complaints are accurate, that their complaints are anchored in love rather than hate, and that it is the way they would love to be treated as well. Always, the use of external whistleblowing should be a last resort.

From the biblical perspective, the good Samaritan went out of his way to assist the wounded stranger. When nurses blow the whistle, they often do so by going out of their way to respond to the required obligation of reporting an unsafe practice. To blow the whistle against a fellow colleague requires tremendous moral courage. Knowing the right thing to do does not necessarily guarantee that one will do the right thing.

Standing up for one's values is an essential aspect of moral courage (Kidder, 2003). Kidder (2003) identified three elements of moral courage as "a commitment to moral principles, an awareness of the dangers involved in supporting those principles and a willing endurance of that danger" (p. 7). There are dangers that come with moral courage in nursing practice, especially, but not exclusively, in the context of whistleblowing. The Christian nurse needs to be aware of these dangers and determined to endure the challenges and obstacles that come from doing the right thing, while relying on the help and grace of God. The pain of not doing anything by the Christian nurse who sees an abusive incident or unsafe nursing practice could even surpass the challenges of whistleblowing.

Evident in the Scriptures are instances where Jesus blew the whistle by courageously calling out on the scribes and pharisees for their hypocrisy. In the gospel of Matthew, Chapter 23, Jesus warned the people about the hypocrisy of the scribes and the pharisees, who liked to be called masters, sit in the public places, and practise their almsgiving in public to get attention. Jesus called them hypocrites simply because their intentions were not sincere, and they often did not practise what they preached. Jesus displayed tremendous moral courage while blowing the whistle and calling out the scribes and the pharisees, who were regarded as powerful people due to their knowledge of the law.

In the gospel of Matthew, Jesus also confronted the chief priests and the scribes when they broke the law by defiling the temple in the context of buying and selling in the temple and making personal profits. Jesus drove out the people who were buying and selling, threw out the tables of money changers and the people who were buying doves, and stated, "My house should be a house of prayer and you are turning it into the den of robbers" (Matthew 21: 12-13). Jesus spoke out bravely and assertively against practices that were not aligned with the right doctrine and what it means to be an authentic Christian.

The Christian nurse must stand up for what is right and fulfill professional obligations by reporting unsafe nursing practices through the channels established in the policies and procedures in their workplace. Keeping the rules and regulations at the workplace, which are meant to keep everyone safe, and preserving the therapeutic milieu of nursing professional practice is equally living according to the will of God. Lastly, it is important that the Christian nurse engage in reflective practice as often as practicable, to make sure that the underlying drive or motivator for all they do is love not hate. Christian nurses must endeavour to ensure that love informs and influences their nursing practice. The love and the respect for the patients, who are the consumers of the nurses' care and service, the love and the respect Christian nurses have for God, for human beings, for nursing, and for themselves, should be the principal motivator. The underlying drive for their whistleblowing, in particular, should be a last resort rather than their first line of nursing intervention when they see unsafe nursing practices and ethical and moral misconduct in their workplace or their organization.

CHAPTER 5: Medication Error

Mistakes are a fact of life.
It is how you respond to error that counts.
—Nikki Giovanni.

THE IDEA OF "do no harm" is the ethical concept that is both fundamental and foundational to nursing professional practice. At the heart of this concept lies the six rights of medication administration in nursing, which are as follows: right patient, right medication, right dose, right time, right route, and right documentation (Rosdahl & Kowalski, 2008). The philosophy behind these rights or checks is to facilitate the enhancement of accuracy during medication administration and to eradicate, or at least minimize, the chances of medication error. The nurse should adopt a personalized strategy that is grounded in the above six checks to further improve accuracy, such as using a calculator to measure the doses of IV and IM medications and double-checking them with a reliable co-worker, who should also confirm the accuracy of the dose by doing their own independent calculation with a calculator. And, as a rule of thumb, the nurse should be asking questions, especially when the physician order appears not to be consistent with their prior knowledge of the medication.

It is a common practice that most physician orders are handwritten. This practice sometimes comes with a problem of illegibility or unreadable handwriting. The nurse should not speculate on what they think the doctor was trying to write or assume what they think the doctor was trying to write. When in doubt, the nurse should not proceed with medication administration. Instead, the nurse should call the physician, clarify the order, and document the clarification. I have seen cases where nurses are afraid to call the physician for fear of incurring their displeasure. This should not be the case. The nurse is an independent practitioner that works collaboratively with the team, just as the physician is. The nurse does not work *for* the physician, at least not in Canada. The nurse works *with* the physician in delivering safe and competent care. And both parties are paid well for the work they do. They are not working for free.

Let us try to put ourselves in the shoes of the patient who is the victim of the nurse's medication error. Imagine a situation where the nurse is the patient who is about to undergo a major surgery, only to learn that they have been injected with a wrong medication, maybe the medication they are allergic to, and now they are having an anaphylactic reaction. A situation such as this can destroy the life of the patient. Also, a situation such as this can mentally and emotionally destroy the nurse who made the medication error; it can terminate the nurse's career and expose them to litigation.

When I was crafting my dissertation in my Ph.D. program, I used a hermeneutic phenomenological approach and interview method to explore the nurses' lived experience of their nursing practice, and one of the nurses who was a participant in that study shared her experience following a medication error. They described medication error as the "dread of every nurse," especially, but not exclusively, due to the dangers that come with medication error.

Nursing is a rewarding career, and most of the people who came to nursing simply want to promote patient's health and help facilitate patients' recovery and wellness. Nevertheless, nursing is as well a demanding career, one that always keeps nurses on their toes and demands a lot of critical thinking. Moreover, with the complexity of patients' medical needs, the number of patients assigned to each nurse, the budget constraints, and the push by the politicians to balance the budget, nurses are frequently exposed to increased workloads, which could translate to increased chances of medication errors.

A study by Cheragi, Manoocheri, Mohammadnejad and Ehsani (2013) found out that medication errors had been made by almost sixty-five percent of the nurses and that the most common type of medication errors for nurses were wrong IV dosage and infusion rate. The authors identified a deficiency in adequate pharmacological knowledge and intervention and the increase in the number of patient load for each nurse as significant causes of medication errors in nursing. The reality and the frequency of medication errors in nursing is well grounded in nursing literature.

It is also a fundamental duty of the nurse to ask critical questions about the medications ordered by the physician, especially regarding the dose of the medication, and to verify orders that appear suspicious for the sake of clarity before administering medication. For the mere fact that a medication was ordered by the physician to be administered by the nurse is not enough reason to absolutely justify the nurse's action of administering erroneous medication.

During clinical practical in nursing school, clinical instructors urged student nurses not to administer any medication they were unfamiliar with, including the side effects of the medication. That is the reason why the clinical instructors often quizzed student nurses about their patient's medications prior to administration. Similar teachings in nursing schools should translate to nursing practices. Nurses have the responsibility to understand both the pharmacokinetics and pharmacodynamics of any medication they are administering. It is the professional responsibility of the nurse to understand the details of any medication before administration, including the medication's contraindications and side effects. The pharmacology courses taken in nursing school should provide the nurse with the entry knowledge about medication administration, including the knowledge of the resources to explore, to facilitate medication administration accuracy. The nurse must understand that just as medication errors happen in nursing, the same is the case with the physician's order. Nurses who administer wrongly ordered medication without having the knowledge of the medication, including the right dose, could also be found to be negligent of their duty.

Apart from the fact that medication error could trigger internal investigation and potential discipline by the employer, it could also trigger a professional investigation by the nursing regulatory bodies and a civil lawsuit by the patient and their family. Depending on many factors, including the nature or the seriousness of the medication error and the frequency of its occurrence from the nurse, the outcome of professional investigations could recommend that the nurse take more pharmacology courses. In some extreme cases, the nurse's licence to practise may be suspended or revoked.

The impact of medication error in nursing practice is huge. Medication error in nursing can lead to the death of a patient and can cause permanent or temporary damage to the individual who is the victim of the nurse's medication error. In extreme cases where death resulted from the nurse's medication error, the impact of such an error can be both traumatic and devastating to the family members of the dead patient. The awareness of the fact that the death of a loved one could have been prevented adds insult to the disastrous experience of the patient's family members, who are mourning the death of a patient. The impact and gravity of shame and guilt that come from medication errors can also be emotionally and mentally devastating to the nurse and could trigger psychological trauma or post-traumatic stress disorder.

So, what would a Christian nurse do after a medication error? It takes humility, honesty, and sincerity to acknowledge and take responsibility for an error, including a medical one. So, the Christian nurse should honestly, humbly, and sincerely acknowledge that they have made a medication error in the first place, and they should not attempt to cover it up to avoid

going through the unpleasant, but necessary, steps in place following a medication error. The Christian nurse should follow
the policy and protocol established in the workplace for
dealing with medication error. Sometimes, in some agencies,
the protocols include a thorough assessment of the patient
involved, notifying the physician on call, following the recom-
mended intervention from the physician on call or from the
facility's standing order, which may include administering a
commonly used medication called Narcan, and a thorough
documentation of the incident.

The Christian nurse should not allow the awful feeling of
failure that comes with medication error to drive them into an
attempt to cover up their mistake. Instead, after following the
reporting protocol established by the workplace, the Christian
nurse should always ask themselves questions such as, "What
did I learn from this awful experience?" and, "What will I do
differently in the future to avoid making a similar mistake?"
Reflective practice facilitates the acquisition of knowledge
about what to do differently, which may include thoroughly
making sure that all the six checks or rights of medication
administration are done prior to giving patients their medication. A mistake of this nature, if processed in a healthy way
and accepted in humility, can positively impact the Christian
nurse's practice and could be a constant reminder about the
need to be meticulous in future medication administration. I
believe that the greatest mistake is the failure to learn from the
past experiences and mistakes and consequently repeating the
same mistake in the future.

John Dewey (1933) was right when he argued persuasively
that we do not necessarily learn from experience, but by

reflecting on our experiences. In other words, insight could be gained through reflective practice. The insight gained from reflective practice could inform and influence the future practice of the Christian nurse. Reflection is an important concept in teaching and learning activities. Reflection promotes one's cognitive awareness and consciousness, and it could help Christian nurses evaluate their practice, which could translate to improved nursing practice competence.

The mistake most Christians and, in our context, Christian nurses make during a difficult time, such as the crisis of medication error, is that they tend to rely only on their human reasoning while abandoning the divine counsel. Often, the Christian nurse is filled with anger while asking some existential questions, such as, "Why did God leave me in this mess? Where is God? Has God abandoned me? My career is over, why call on God now?" These are genuine questions. It shows how we feel. It becomes a conscious reminder that we are still human. But the truth is that God is usually closest to us during those trying times, including the times when we feel that He is far from us. It takes a leap of faith and a total surrender to the will and the providence of God.

I, therefore, admonish the Christian nurse to meticulously do all the six medication checks/rights prior to medication administration, regardless of how busy the workplace and the patient load is. I encourage the Christian nurse to apply moral courage and to do what is right in the event of medication error by following the reporting, assessment, and intervention protocols in place in their workplace. It is a statement of fact that medication error is the "dread of every nurse." Nevertheless, do not allow the rigorous and unpleasant, but necessary, process of reporting medication error move you toward a cover-up. Lastly, remember that God is closest to you during unpleasant, stressful, and challenging times, and that God will make a way where there seems to be none. Nothing is impossible to God. Sometimes, everything may not necessarily go the way you plan. Remember, God knows the best!

CHAPTER 6: Therapeutic Communication With the Patient

*Life doesn't make any sense without
interdependence. We need each other, and the
sooner we learn that, the better for us all.*
—Erik Erikson

THERAPEUTIC COMMUNICATION IS an interaction that happens between a patient and the nurse with the aim of improving the physical and the emotional wellbeing of the patient. It is a thoughtful conversation between the patient and the nurse, which is grounded in mutual respect, trust, and acceptance, and it encourages patients to express their opinions and feelings in a safe and therapeutic environment. Therapeutic communication is central to competent nursing, and it helps the nurse establish therapeutic rapport with patients. It is an active listening where nurses immerse themselves in the narrative and the story of patients to thoroughly understand and assess patients' needs, with the intention of planning interventions that are specific to those needs, and provide patient and family-centred care.

One of the prominent features of nurse-patient therapeutic communication is that it is usually tailored and suited around patients' needs. In other words, it should be particular and relevant to the needs of the patient and their family. As a professional communication, it requires that nurses maintain professional distance and boundaries during the conversation, while at the same time immersing themselves in the narrative and the story of the patient, trying to understand patients' needs as patients perceive them. By immersing themselves in the narratives of the patient through active listening, nurses could obtain insight into the core values and beliefs of the patient, including the patient's illness experience and their religious and cultural beliefs, to integrate those fundamental values and belief systems into the patient's care plan.

The concepts of cultural sensitivity and cultural awareness are central to understanding patients' ways of life, values, beliefs, and what is pertinent to patients. Cultural sensitivity enables the nurse to understand, accept, and be consciously aware of patients' culture, with the knowledge that no culture is intrinsically wrong when perceived through the lens of the original and authentic citizens of that culture. Cultural sensitivity could help the nurse understand the differences between their own values and beliefs from those of the patient. If there are differences between the nurse and the patient, they do not need to be reconciled during therapeutic communication with the patient because reconciliation of cultural values and beliefs is not the goal of nurse-patient therapeutic communication. It is important that nurses evaluate their personal values and beliefs, including their biases, to control them, making sure that they don't interfere with their patient's care.

Therapeutic communication is anchored in knowledge and constructive emotion. The information and assessment that the nurse provides should be grounded in empirical knowledge. Constructive emotion, especially in the context of empathy, is an indispensable component of nursing therapeutic conversations with the patient. The idea of empathy is better explained and understood in the context of role-playing. This role-playing implies that nurses should immerse themselves in the experience and narrative of the patient to fully understand how the patient feels and view reality through their lens.

Nurses' therapeutic communications with patients require skills and techniques to facilitate patients' expression of feelings and ideas. It is a communication that requires an active listening to what the client is saying, which means that the nurse should stay with the topic that is important to the patient, while being consciously aware of both the verbal and non-verbal cues. While immersed in the patient's story, the nurse should aim to establish a rapport, which could help the nurse to share observations, clarify ideas, restate the ideas using their words, offer empathy and feelings, offer hope, provide information that is grounded in knowledge, and, lastly, summarize the information received from the patient, which gives the patient the sense of confidence that the information they relayed was accurately absorbed by the nurse.

So much information is obtained through this conversation. Through therapeutic conversation, the nurse can identify the patient's risks and problems, which could provide the nurse with teaching opportunity around diseases prevention and health promotion. Therapeutic conversation facilitates nursing planning, intervention, and evaluation of the effectiveness of the action taken by the nurse in response to the needs presented by the patient. Often, patients come to the hospital with complex needs, such as physical needs, psychological needs, emotional needs and spiritual needs. It is a fundamental lack when the nurse is incapable of assessing the needs of the patients in any of these areas. How and what, then, would a Christian nurse do in order to engage in effective therapeutic communication with patients and thereby provide competent assessments and interventions that are both specific and patient-centred?

First, the Christian nurse should strive to acquire the necessary nursing communication skills that translate to effective and therapeutic nursing communication, such as active listening, sharing empathy, using humour, knowing when it is appropriate to use touch and silence, and offering hope, to mention but a few. These skills are essential components of competent therapeutic communication because they encourage and facilitate patients' expression of feelings and ideas. The Christian nurse should always remember that therapeutic communication is mutually shared, and it is a two-way process and technique, where both parties listen and give each other the opportunity to talk.

Second, the Christian nurse should endeavour to ground the information they are giving to patients on empirical nursing knowledge and nursing best practice guidelines, which is consistent with the practice guideline in their workplace. Also, the Christian nurse should always remember that their role in the clinical practice is nursing to everyone. During a spiritual assessment of the patient's needs, for example, the Christian nurse should not be afraid to respond if the patient is interested, willing, and proactively starts the discussion on God and beliefs in the existence of supernatural reality or spirituality, especially if this is relevant to the patient's recovery and it acts as a coping mechanism. Be careful not to give patients false hope. Be conscious of the reality of delusions of religious type. The Christian nurse should be careful not to affirm or enable delusional thought content. Be willing to explore and address false beliefs in a non-confrontational manner and prompt the patient toward accurate or right information.

Remember that science and religion, faith and reason, although very distinct, are not mutually exclusive in nursing clinical practice. Remember to ask patients whether they would like follow-up resources available through the hospital or the facility's chaplain, if applicable. Remember that nursing is your primary role in the clinical setting, and nursing is a regulated practice. Remember that your primary role is not the chaplain's role. Remember that therapeutic communication is not necessarily an opportunity to preach the gospel of Christ or to convert the unbelievers. It is not an opportunity for evangelization, per se. But Christian nurses can make meaningful impact on the patients by their actions and by the way they nurse, for actions speak louder than words.

During therapeutic communication with the patient, the Christian nurse should be consciously aware of the need to be "quick to listen, slow to speak, and slow to become angry" as evident in the epistle of James chapter one, verse 19. The Christian nurse should not pretend to know everything or have answers to all the patients' questions. The Christian nurse needs humility, honesty, and genuineness to be able to say that they do not know or have the answer to the question. The Christian nurse should notify the patient that they will consult the care team and present the question to the team, and they should explore other necessary resources, if applicable, with a plan to provide meaningful feedback to the patient regarding the question asked by the patient.

As a Christian nurse, have you ever been in a situation where a patient asked you to pray with them or for them? What was your response? What is your facility's guideline on this situation? What should the Christian nurse do? I firmly believe that every situation is context-specific, and context is important in any assessment and intervention. First, it is completely appropriate for a Christian nurse to pray for, and pray with, the patient if they make this request, as long as this request is not initiated by the Christian nurse. It is also important for the Christian nurse to clarify with patients what they would like the nurse to pray for, without making unnecessary assumptions. The goal here is to meet the needs of patients and not to meet what the nurse thinks the patient should need.

The Christian nurse's therapeutic communication with patients, given the appropriate context, and when it is rightfully requested and initiated by patients, can include praying with patients, in line with the idea of meeting patients' needs in holistic context. The Christian nurse should pray with the patient in a way that is fitting and that aligns with the nurse's and the patient's spiritual belief, without making any party uncomfortable, and in accordance with the workplace guidelines.

The Christian nurse should align their practice with the philosophy of servant leadership model, with the primary aim of caring for, and serving, the needs of patients first. And, through service, the Christian nurse should proceed to lead in praying for the needs of patients, in advocating for patients, and in teaching patients about health promotions and disease prevention, for example, while grounding the information that is relayed to patients in evidence-based nursing best practices.

The qualities of servant leadership, such as empathy, listening, stewardship, and commitment to the growth of the people (Spears, 2010), to mention but a few, are qualities that should be at the heart of every Christian nurse. The qualities of servant leadership model encourage holistic approach to nursing care and nursing leadership, and, as such, advance qualities that are both fundamental and foundational to competent nursing practice (Onwuegbuchunam, 2020).

Empathy, an essential quality of servant leadership, should be central to the heart and practice of a Christian nurse. Servant leaders make sincere and conscious effort to understand and empathize with others (Spears, 2010). With empathy, the servant leader (the nurse) makes conscious effort to stand in other peoples' shoes and attempt to understand and view reality from the point of view of others (Northouse, 2013). Servant leaders make honest efforts to understand the illness experiences of their clients through the application of constructive emotion. The application of empathy and regulated emotion in the Christian nurse's therapeutic conversation with the patient could translate to effective nursing communication that is relevant, specific, and patient-centred.

Listening is an essential quality of a servant leader. Servant leaders seek to understand and address the needs of their clients by being open-minded and validating what is being said and unsaid, by listening to their inner voices, and by engaging in reflective practice (Spears, 2010). Servant leaders begin their communication by actively listening first, and responding to any problem or to any issue raised, after listening as a matter of priority (Greenleaf, 1991). Through listening support, servant leaders validate the opinions and emotions of their patients to align their interventions with the needs of their clients. A Christian nurse in the clinical setting should strive to develop a habit of listening to patients with rapt attention to appropriately respond to their needs. The importance of developing listening ears was underscored in the Bible, especially, but not exclusively, in the call of Samuel (1 Samuel 3: 7-11). The Christian nurse should always pray for listening ears to understand the needs of their patients, which will then inform their nursing interventions.

Stewardship is an important trait of servant leaders. Servant leaders are stewards who are engaged and devoted to serving the needs of others (Spears, 2010). Stewardship is understood in the context of taking responsibility for the role entrusted to the leader. Servant leaders accept the duty and commitment to serve and care for the people and the organization entrusted to their care (Northouse, 2013). Christian nurses should always treat their patients as partners because the information that patients provide is crucial in planning competent intervention, with the knowledge that it is the responsibility they owe to the patients entrusted to their care, and in meeting the needs of the health care organization in general.

Commitment to the growth of the people (Spears, 2010) is another quality of a servant leader that every Christian nurse should always aspire to possess. Servant leaders operate with the mindset that each individual is unique and has an intrinsic value beyond their material contributions to the organization (Spears, 2010). The Christian nurse in the clinical setting should always bear in mind that they are working because the patients are in their workplace in the first place, and without the patients, their presence as nurses may not be needed. This mindset will help the Christian nurse put the needs of patients first and commit to the healing, growth, and wellbeing of all the patients entrusted to their care.

CHAPTER 7: **Punctuality and Duty of Care**

Want of punctuality is a want of virtue.
—John M. Mason

PUNCTUALITY AND DUTY of care are two essential aspects central to competent nursing practice. The role of the nurse is so critical because it is directly connected with the health and life of the people. The duty and actions of the nurse could positively or negatively impact the greatest possession of humans: the life of the people. Due to the nature of the nurse's work, it is therefore both legally and ethically imperative that nurses understand the seriousness of the duty of care and punctuality in their practice, as well as the notion that lateness to work and negligence is almost inexcusable in any circumstance.

Nursing work is a teamwork. The nurse works independently and collaboratively with other health care professionals to provide health services to patients. The nurse who demonstrates a habit of lateness to work is directly or indirectly negatively impacting the whole team members, including the team dynamic and morale. The negative vibes from the nurse's lateness to work also has negative impact on the quality of care that patients receive. The nurse's lateness to work is a complete disservice to the rest of the team, who must often work together and whose work is somewhat interdependent and interconnected with what each member of the team does.

The situation of nurses who work in intensive care units, psychiatry in-patient units, and medical emergency departments, including psychiatry emergency departments, is a practical example to concretely demonstrate how the nurse's lateness to work can negatively impact other members of the team. Due to the high patient acuity that is often associated with these departments, it becomes unsafe to leave patients uncared for, or unattended to, at any given time. But the lateness of a nurse to work for shift report and handover often results in a decrease in care. Other nurses who have done their due diligence at work for their shift could be exposed and forced to extend their work hours or to work mandatory overtime, for example, due to the tardiness of another nurse. Nursing could be mentally, emotionally, and physically exhausting, and being forced to work extra time when the nurse is not psychologically, cognitively, and physically prepared for the extension could trigger unpleasant feelings among the team, and negatively impact the staff morale.

Nursing work is considered an essential service. Often, when nurses are forced or mandated to work overtime, it has direct negative impact on the quality of care that patients receive. Humans function at their optimal level when they are well rested, and have enough energy. The same is the case in nursing. Nurses function better when they are not tired. When the quality of care that patients receive is negatively impacted, it also compromises the safety of the patient, and it exposes them to dangers, such as medication error.

Nursing facilities, including hospitals, are open for twenty-four hours per day, seven days a week, and they operate through shift work. Those of us who have worked night shifts in the hospital at some point in our career know how the nurse who was up for the whole night is more than ready to give the shift report and run home to sleep. It becomes a nightmare and a huge risk to tell that nurse to extend their shift for one or two hours more because the day shift nurse who was supposed to take over the care of patients will be late. To say the least, from my experience, it was not fun. The night nurse is therefore being exposed to huge risks and liabilities because nursing work requires a lot of critical thinking that demands the nurse's physical, cognitive, mental, and emotional capacities to be working at the optimal level.

Punctuality is anchored in respect. Punctuality has to do with respect for time and respect for others, which, in nursing practice, extends to include respect for people's lives. Punctuality in nursing practice is a demonstration of good character, and it is compulsorily important for good nursing practice (Helmstadter & Godden, 2013). For the Christian nurse, punctuality and duty of care should be perceived and understood as essential qualities and ways to demonstrate the love for people, which implies showing great respect for people's lives, a demonstration of discipline, a respect for time, and a possession of good moral character.

I contend that tardiness has no place in nursing professional practice, and that punctuality is a demonstration of one's sense of accountability and responsibility. For the Christian nurse, to be punctual in the workplace implies that the nurse is mentally, physically, spiritually, and cognitively prepared to be present in the moment, without any interruption, mental distractions, or disturbances. It is the nurse's full commitment to the care and service of patients as a priority and the self-immersion of the nurse into the wellbeing of patients without any reservation.

The duty of care, on the other hand, is the professional obligation of every nurse. As a matter of fact, the duty of care in nursing practice is the obligation or responsibility that demands that nurses totally act in the best interest of patients, while making sure that their own personal interests do not impede or conflict with their nursing duty. Caring is central and foundational to nursing. The duty of care comprised of the legal, ethical, and professional rules and regulations that are in place to protect patients from injury or harm while they are under the care of a nurse. The duty of care also exposes the nurse to legal and disciplinary actions if breached (Water, Rasmussen, Neufeld, Gerrard & Ford, 2017). Nurses are obligated to care for the patients by the nature of their work, and nurses are endowed with the duty of care, which demands that they should do no harm to the people entrusted to their care. The duty of care in nursing practice is grounded in the principle of non-maleficence and beneficence.

The concept of duty of care highlights the fact that negligence of duty comes with liability. Smith and Keatings (2000) identified three essential components that must be present to establish a case of negligence: an individual had a duty of care to the other; an individual failed to fulfil or to carryout the duty owed to the other; and, lastly, harm or damage was caused to the other. Since nurses are entrusted with the obligation to care for the public, which implies having a duty of care to the public, nurses are also held accountable for any injury or damage caused to the patients, whether intentional or unintentional, in the process of caring for the patients. Nurses' errors, such as in the administration of medication or persistent lateness to work, can cause harm to the patient and expose the nurse to legal, ethical, and professional reprimand.

It is the professional responsibility of the nurse to provide safe and competent care that accounts for patients' perceptions and opinions and is anchored in respecting the patient's wishes. The nurse has a professional duty to fully give patients the information they need to make informed decisions about their care, in the context of respecting patients' right to autonomy and empowering patients to take ownership of their health. The nurse also has to be consciously aware that while it is necessary to respect patients' wishes and opinions and incorporate them in the care they provide, those wishes have to align with, or at least not conflict with, the guidelines set by the nursing regulatory bodies and nursing best practices.

The nursing professional's duty to care for patients entails that nurses should not provide any care that could expose the patients to unreasonable risks, with the knowledge that providing such care could implicate the nurse in professional reprimands and legal litigation. Equally important is the need for the nurse to constantly engage in reflective practice and be consciously aware of their prejudices, biases, and personal opinions on patients' worldviews, cultures, or even lifestyles, in order to control them and to make sure that those personal opinions and values do not impede or compromise the care they provide.

The Christian nurse, therefore, must be cognizant of the concepts of duty of care and sense of duty while caring for the patients. The Christian nurse's sense of duty extends to include the desire to perceive nursing work as an opportunity to serve God and the patients entrusted to their care just as Jesus did, with patience and humility, even during a difficult day. Christian nurses should do their best to present themselves to work as nurses who are both competent and eager to serve the people entrusted to their care, while being fully aware of the advice of St. Paul to the Colossians, "whatever you do, work at it with all your heart, as working for the Lord, not for human masters" (Col. 3:23). This advice is significant. It is both informative and transformative. If Christian nurses understand that their work, which is financially rewarding, could also be an opportunity to serve both God and humans, it will transform their practice. And, with this knowledge, it could be easier for the Christian nurse to persevere in any challenge they encounter at their workplace. The same work that is an opportunity for making a rewarding and an honest living could also be an opportunity for salvation, and a source of blessings from God to the patients.

Christian nurses should perceive themselves as the stewards of the patients and work very hard to demonstrate competence and accountability in their care of the patients. Jesus often used parables in his teachings, especially while illustrating the ideas of dignity of labour, sense of duty, stewardship, and hard work. In the parable of the talents evident in the gospels of Matthew, Chapter 25 and Luke, Chapter 19, respectively, Jesus told the story of a master who placed his servants in charge of his business while he was away for a significant time, probably in order to assess their hard work, sense of duty, and stewardship. When the master returned from the trip, he assessed their performance according to how faithfully, productively, and hard they worked to obtain profit with the goods entrusted to their care. The master rewarded each of the servants who demonstrated great sense of duty and worked assiduously as good steward. The unfaithful servant, who did not work hard, was negatively compensated.

These parables have always resonated with me personally in my nursing professional practice, especially in the context of the necessity and the relevancy that Christian nurses should be good stewards to the clients entrusted to their care. There is always an assessment of nursing practice. The assessment could come from your clients, your supervisors, or your colleagues. Feedback, both constructive and destructive, is evident in nursing practice. Also, in nursing practice, every nurse keeps an eye on the practice of the other, either directly or indirectly, primarily to ensure that safe care is provided to the patients. Every nurse has an opinion about other nurses. There is always that subterranean judgment and assessment of each nurse's performance. The Christian nurse should remember that Jesus also used parables to show the relevancy of assessment and judgment when one is entrusted with something—in nurses' case, patients' lives. Therefore, the Christian nurse ought to be consciously aware of St. Paul's advice to Timothy to "do your best to present yourself to God as one approved, a worker who does not need to be ashamed and who correctly handles the word of truth." Here, the word of truth in your nursing practice quickly becomes the message you spread through your actions and how you care for the people God has entrusted to your care, in line with the guidelines for nursing professional practice. Indeed, actions speak louder than words, and the message of truth can be spread in your workplace by your actions, for by their fruits you will know them (Matthew 7:20).

The Christian nurse should remember that as Christians in general, we are required to care for and love one another. The Christian's call to care and love one another should be the underlying drive for the Christian nurse to display an exceptional sense of duty to care for their patients. It should be the underlying motivator and the internal drive for the Christian nurse to be punctual and to be mentally, spiritually, emotionally, and physically prepared and presentable to care for patients, to go extra miles when needed, and to elevate their nursing professional practice.

CHAPTER 8: Self-Care and Avoiding Burnout

Come to me all you that labour and are loaded
with burdens, and I will give you rest.
—Matthew 11:28

BURNOUT IS A central issue in nursing professional practice that is well documented in nursing literature and commonly experienced by many nurses, as a matter of fact. Nurses work around the clock, both in the hospital settings and in designated care centres, which are complex work environments that require a lot of critical thinking, continuous assessment, and continuous intervention. In these environments, nurses' work can be both cognitively and emotionally demanding and challenging.

Nurses' complex workplace is filled with traumas, deaths, pain, complex physical health conditions, and psychological issues, which often impact the nurses' own mental and physical health, both directly and indirectly, and could translate to burnout. It becomes a double tragedy when the environment in which nurses work is toxic, untherapeutic, oppressive, and unsupportive of nurses' work and the issues that they bring forward to the employers, especially regarding their mental and physical health. When nurses feel that their voices are not heard and that the management is not very supportive, it could lead to dissatisfaction with their work, and that could translate to burnout.

Most care facilities are called nursing units because the work of the nurse is central to the wellbeing of the patients. Nursing care is often twenty-four-hour care, involving shift work and weekends. As such, nurses have great knowledge of patients' conditions in holistic contexts. Nurses are with the patients throughout their illness and recovery journeys. Nurses see the patients in their most vulnerable times, and they see the patients in their happy moments after recovery. Nurses are the advocates of the patients, and nurses participate in leading change and creating visions for the health care system. When employers fail to listen to the vital contribution of the nurse to the health care team, it could be discouraging to the nurse, and it could make nurses to feel that their work is not valued. These negative feelings could lead to compassion fatigue, which is a situation where the nurse experiences emotional, mental, and physical exhaustion that translates to diminished ability to empathize or relate to patients with compassion.

Burnout in nursing is explained in the context of continuous and persistent exposure to a physically and emotionally stressful workplace, which makes the nurse feel challenged, overwhelmed, exhausted, self-doubtful, angry, anxious, inadequate, and inefficient (Maslach & Leiter, 2005). This cognitive and emotional exhaustion is evident in nursing burnout, and it could translate to a situation where nurses lack a sense of accomplishment and fail to find meaning in what they do. This fundamental lack negatively impacts the nurses' confidence and effectiveness, and it negatively impacts the quality of care that patients receive.

There are many factors that can contribute to burnout in nursing. As a matter of fact, burnout usually happens as a result of extremely intense and mismanaged stress. Acute stress or prolonged stress is the leading factor that contributes to burnout in nursing. Stress is part of life. We have healthy stress that motivates us to accomplish things or respond to our activities of daily living. This type of stress is often manageable, and it does not necessarily lead to burnout. But improperly managed stress, especially stress that is acute, extreme, and prolonged, leads to a burnout, and this type of stress is both physically and mentally damaging to the nurse.

Another factor that could lead to burnout in nursing is the increase in the workload that nurses are expected to complete on every shift. Health science is always in flux. Events that happen in a care facility, especially tragic events, are often investigated, which leads to recommendations to prevent its reoccurrence. This makes perfect sense. But nurses often find themselves in situations with ever-increasing recommendations and additions to the tasks they are expected to complete, without anything being removed from the previous lists of tasks they are expected to accomplish, and without an increase in the staffing baseline. The situation is even worse where the care facility is a private health care institution that is for profit. More often than not, in these facilities, everything anchors on the bottom line, and if something is not financially expedient, it is usually not the top priority. Over time, this increase in nurses' workloads could make nurses feel the heat of compassion fatigue and burnout.

Lack of a supportive workplace environment could cause fatigue in the nurse. When nurses feel that their concerns, opinions, and emotions are not supported and validated by the employer, they can feel powerless, and they can experience a total disconnect from the management and other health care teams. This situation could cause crises and a lack of belonging for the nurse. It could negatively impact the nurse's performance and mental health, and it could lead to burnout and dissatisfaction.

Most of the people that came to nursing sincerely want to help patients get better and make a difference in the community where they practise. Sometimes, however, the organizational values are distant and distinct from the values and visions that nurses firmly hold, especially with regard to giving competent care; when those values are sacrificed at the altar of the bottom line, it could trigger job dissatisfaction to the nurse. In this type of situation, nurses are therefore left to practise against the values they firmly hold. This situation could translate to burnout. Having said that, rendering quality care and profit are not mutually exclusive.

Besides, with the increase in the workload of the nurse and the stressful demands of nursing job, nurses sometimes find themselves in situations where they are not compensated well for the work they do and the wealth of knowledge they possess. Given the nursing profession's emphasis on the continuing competence of the nurse, many nurses aspire to maximize their knowledge and enhance their credentials, which some employers do not recognize and do not reward. Highly competent nurses unsupportive environments where the employer does not appreciate their worth, and where there is little or no opportunity for reward and promotion, could feel less valued, frustrated, and dissatisfied. These negative feelings could eventually lead to burnout.

Self-Care

The idea of maintaining a balance between hard work and self-care is foundational to competent nursing practice, and it is central to healthy lifestyle. Nurses are in care and service industries that are often fast paced and demand a lot of critical thinking. Nurses often encounter situations where they have to work long hours or skip their breaks to meet the needs and the care of patients, which they perceive to be a matter of priority. A self-care deficit can negatively impact the physical, emotional, mental, and spiritual wellbeing of the nurse, and it could lead to compassion fatigue and burnout. It is a well-documented fact that burnout in nursing also has huge repercussions on the quality of care that patients receive and the health care system as a whole. To reduce or eliminate dissatisfaction and burnout in nursing, self-care is necessary for health and wellness.

Nurses function at their optimal level when they attend to their personal health needs and perceive their self-care as central to their ability to function competently. Nurses' self-care not only helps them advance their own health and wellness, but also to advance and promote the quality of care that patients receive and the safety of the patients under their care.

Self-care is grounded in both knowledge and action. Self-care highlights the need for self-knowledge and self-awareness. Self-care is to be perceived and understood within the holistic health and well-being of nurses, where the nurse invests and is invested in maintaining a healthy balance between their cognitive, affective, mental, and spiritual well-being. Self-care involves all the knowledge and deliberate actions that the nurse takes to improve their health, maintain equilibrium in life, and decrease stress and anxiety.

Self-care in nursing is often overlooked by majority of nurses. But the importance of self-care among nurses is crucial because it is related to both the health of the nurse and the health of the patients under the nurse's care. The rationale here is that a lack of self-care by the nurse affects their level of functionality and the quality of care they provide to the patients. Self-care in nursing does not imply selfishness in any way. Rather, it is an expression of knowledge, a sense of responsibility and accountability, and the duty that nurses owe to their own health. To effectively take care of the other, the nurse must maintain a balanced lifestyle with the knowledge and awareness that health is understood in holistic context. Self-care refuels and rejuvenates the nurse to care for the patients effectively.

Central to the importance of self-care in nursing practice is the nurse's personalized assessment of their self-care deficits in the areas of physical, spiritual, mental, and emotional wellbeing, since health is understood holistically, in order to plan interventions that are relevant to their needs and effective as well. These personal assessments by the nurse could help the nurse identify and explore avenues and opportunities for growth. The physical needs of the nurse could include activities such as eating well, exercising, and weight management. The mental needs of the nurse may include using relaxation techniques and practising mindfulness. Their spiritual needs may require that nurses reconnect with nature, reflect on the meaning and purpose of their lives, reflect on their relationship with God and their prayer life, and reconnect with religious groups. The list continues.

Similar to patients' care, every plan, action, and intervention by the nurse, is often followed with an evaluation of the intervention to identify what worked and what did not, and thereby determine what to do differently. In setting their self-care goals, nurses should remember to utilize the commonly used SMART goal acronym (specific, measurable, attainable, realistic and time specific) to plan for a successful outcome. Nurses need to evaluate the actions they take toward their self-care and reflect on their progress to determine whether adjustments are needed.

How, then, will the Christian nurse respond to the issue of burnout and the need for self-care in professional nursing? Evident in the Christian context and the Christian worldview is the belief that the human life is the greatest gift we received from God, and that human beings are the custodian of their lives. To be a good custodian of one's life entails that one must take all the necessary steps to nurture, protect, and preserve oneself in being. I submit that one of the fundamental causes of compassion fatigue and burnout in nursing practice is lack of adequate self-care by the nurse.

The Christian nurse should operate with the mindset that to usefully and competently care for the needs of their patients, the nurse should learn how to care and serve themselves first. This statement does not suggest selfishness on the part of the Christian nurse. Rather, the statement is grounded in knowledge that a healthy nurse with a healthy mind is the one who could better care for, and serve patients.

To maintain a healthy lifestyle in a holistic context that includes physical, spiritual, mental, and emotional health, and thereby function at the optimal level, the Christian nurse should develop healthy strategies to help manage stress and improve health. Strategies may include maintaining a healthy diet, daily exercise, resting or getting a good night's sleep, taking vacations, having a quiet time to meditate, pray, and reflect, spending time with the loved ones, and making out time to appreciate nature, etc. Each of these strategies could rejuvenate and revitalize the Christian nurse; they could help reduce or prevent the chances of burnout, and they could translate to effective nursing care of patients.

Although the need for self-care was not explicitly addressed in the Bible, there are several passages where the need for self-care was implied and expanded. Evident in the book of Exodus, Chapter 34:21, God commanded humans to rest when he asserted: "six days you shall labour, but on seventh day you shall rest; even during the plowing season and harvest you must rest." God himself valued the need for rest as evidenced in the story of creation in the book of Genesis chapter 2:2, where God rested on the seventh after completing the work of creation.

In the New Testament, Jesus also valued the need for self-care and was seen to often withdraw from the crowd after the fatigue of His daily work for quietness, meditation, and prayer in the context of rejuvenation and revitalization of the mind and the body. This assertion finds its vindication in the gospel of Luke 5:16, which states that "Jesus often withdrew to lonely places and prayed." The importance of reflection in nursing cannot be overemphasized. The Christian nurse could gain insight through hindsight, just as Jesus often did, by removing themselves from all the noise and distractions, including technology and friends; they could do this occasionally, when necessary, and as a way of life.

The Christian nurse should always remember that Jesus is the source of true rest, true peace, and true joy. As such, Jesus said: "come to me all you that labour and are loaded with burdens, and I will give you rest" (Matthew 11:28).

It is necessary for the Christian nurse to be consciously aware of the frailty of human nature and the need for human dependence on God. As dependent rational beings, Christian nurses should be consciously aware of their physical and mental limitations and stressors. They should understand that when they care for their minds and bodies, when they eat healthily, exercise daily, and make sure that they are well rested, they are being good stewards of the gift of life (mind and body) that God has given them. Maintaining adequate self-care could make Christian nurses better prepared to serve and care for their patients, better serve God, and help them to prevent or reduce the chances of compassion fatigue and nursing burnout.

The Christian nurse should remember the agape love that Jesus demonstrated on the cross for us; they should remember that God sends His only son to suffer and die for us out of love for our salvation. Since Jesus showed us such a great love and cared for us, I contend that the least we can do as children of God is to love ourselves, take care of ourselves, and take care of the life that God has given us in the context of self-care. Evident in the gospel of Mark 12:31, Jesus commanded us to "love your neighbour as you love yourself." Which implied that Jesus wants us to love ourselves, and the best way to demonstrate that love for ourselves is through self-care. Of course, we are expected to love our neighbour as ourselves. In the context of nursing practice, the greatest neighbour that the nurse has is the patient that is entrusted to their care. In other words, when nurses love themselves and take care of themselves, they will present themselves to work, better prepared in a holistic context to care for the patients, to serve the patients' needs, and to love the patients, who are their neighbours, the way they love themselves.

Jesus was asked a question in the parable of Good Samaritan by an expert in the law" "Who is my neighbour?" Jesus' answer to this question was brilliant, fascinating, and significant. Jesus located and positioned what it means to be a good neighbour to others within the context of practical Christianity, which is anchored in compassion, love, genuine care, and sacrifice. At the end of the parable of the Good Samaritan, Jesus admonished, "go therefore and do likewise" (Luke 10:37).

Often, nurses encounter patients that are wounded physically, emotionally, mentally, and spiritually. The Christian nurse should remember to be a good neighbour to these patients by loving them through their exceptional attitude toward patient care. The nurse should also remember that when they take care of themselves through adequate self-care, they are preparing themselves to competently care for their patients, which, by extension, implies that they are loving their neighbours as themselves.

CHAPTER 9: Grounding Nursing Practice in Prayer

Do not be anxious about anything, but in
every situation, by prayer and petition, with
thanksgiving, present your request to God.
—Philippians 4:5

HUMAN BEINGS ARE unique, and our uniqueness is in plural. Human beings are composed of body and soul, matter and form. The soul, therefore, is considered to be the spiritual component of human persons—the one that yearns for the transcendental being or the metaphysical reality. In his *Confession*, St. Augustine of Hippo asserted that the human soul is restless until it rests in the Lord. This idea of humans as composed beings serves as the philosophical and theological foundation that echoes the importance of spirituality in human life.

Prayer is one of the ways we express our yearnings and our connection with the supernatural being, which, in the Christian context, is God. Christians have always resorted to prayer anchored in faith as a credible means of communication with God, especially, but not exclusively, during difficult times such as sickness and hardship, hoping to receive help and relief from their difficulties. Since spirituality is central to the very nature of humans and prayer is one of the ways to express that natural yearnings for the supernatural being, prayer therefore occupies an essential place in the life of Christians in general and should occupy a vital place in the life of the Christian nurse in particular.

Prayer has been explained and understood as communication with the divine and cosmic deities, whereby spiritual relationship is established (Baesler, 2003). When Christians engage in prayer, they express their recognition and the awareness of their need and dependency on God, who is the only self-subsistent being, while being fully aware that humans are dependent beings. Christians have always looked up to God in prayer, with the hope that their help will come from God, who made heaven and earth (Psalm 124:8).

During the time of stress, burnout, misfortune, hopelessness, and helplessness, Christians often call on God through prayer, with faith and hope that God will soothe the pain and alleviate the crisis. Prayer therefore offers a sense of meaning, identity, and belonging to Christians, and it occupies a central position in the Christian worldview.

Nursing is a profession that is highly demanding, stressful, and rewarding. Nurses' work is complex, and it is done in environments that are often very challenging and require constant critical thinking and alertness. This underscores the need for Christian nurses to form the habit of praying at all times for themselves, for their nursing practice, and for the recovery of their patients. There is evidence that suggests a strong positive correlation between prayer and work-related mental health (Turton & Francis, 2007). Prayer should therefore be a habit and a way of life for the Christian nurse.

Evident in the gospel of Matthew is an invitation from Jesus to all, and in our context, to nurses who are experiencing compassion fatigue and burnout to "come to me all you who are weary and burned, and I will give you rest" (Matthew 11:28). This invitation from Jesus to come to Him through prayer should be a reliable and a credible self-care strategy for the Christian nurse. Also, evident in the Letter of St. James in the New Testament is the following advice: "Is anyone among you in trouble? Let them pray. Is anyone happy? Let them sing songs of praise" (James 5:13).

Equally important is the nurses' practice of presenting to God in prayer whatever they experience in their different workplaces. The Christian nurse should always be grateful to God in the first place for the gift of a good job that pays well, the opportunity to make positive impact in the lives of the people, and the opportunity to bear witness to God primarily through the way they nurse. All the good experiences, challenges, champions, and detractors from workplace should also be placed in the hands of God through prayer, remembering the advice of Jesus to "love your enemies, and pray for those who persecute you" (Matthew 5:44). It is tempting for humans to love only those who love them back and hate those who persecute them. But a call to live a Christian life is a call to love unconditionally, a call to follow the footsteps of Christ.

Christian nurses should also guard against becoming hyper-vigilant, hypersensitive, and suspicious of everyone and everything that happens at the workplace. If they believe that everything has an underlying or subterranean meaning, they easily perceive provocation even when there is no evidence to support such perception and belief. Sometimes, some nurses can cause aggression to other nurses in the workplace. But care should be taken not to confuse constructive feedback, for example, with negativity.

When the Christian nurse prays, it is necessary for the nurse to be flexible with how, when, and what they are asking of God in prayer, and not to be discouraged if the prayer seemed not to have been answered. Remember that God is all loving and all-knowing, and He will always want the best for His children. Remember that God's time and human's time are usually different. Also, it is a common belief that God's time is the best, since God can see the future. Patience, flexibility, and perseverance in prayer are equally important.

The Christian nurse needs to develop a personal relationship with God, a relationship that is anchored in faith and total dependence on God's grace, balanced with honest effort of the nurse to live a life of witness. The nurse should see God as a loving father and a friend. It is a fundamental flaw for the Christian nurse to perceive God as avenging and to believe that He is merely watching to find fault with human beings in order to render punishment and reward good behaviour. The nurse's relationship with God should be grounded in mutual love, with the knowledge that God is always faithful, and that

His love is unconditional. This healthy perception of God should enable the Christian nurse to come to God through prayer in any circumstance, without being afraid of incurring God's displeasure, and with the knowledge that to keep oneself away from God is to be severed from the very source of happiness, rest, love, and peace.

There are several prayer strategies and ways of expressing ourselves to God. In prayer of praise, worship, and adoration, we focus on praising God, reflecting on the greatness of God, and exalting the name of God. We also remember the frail nature of human beings and express our dependence on the grace of God, who is the source and the author of everything that is good. In the prayer of petition, we make our needs known to God in humility, faith, and hope. We ask God to provide for our spiritual and material needs, we submit our experiences in the workplace, and in life in general, to God, while asking God to grant our requests. In the end, we submit our petitions, hopes, and ambitions to the will of God, asking for God's will to be done in our lives, for indeed, it is only in the will of God that we are free. The prayer of intercession is primarily where we pray for various needs. It is where we pray for colleagues at work, for example—both champions and detractors. It is where we pray for our family members, our patients, and others who asked us to keep them in our prayers. In the prayer of thanksgiving, we express our gratitude to God for the things that he has done in our lives, and for the blessings we have received from Him. We also thank Him for the things that he is yet to do.

Jesus gave us an example of how to pray in the famous prayer called "The Lord's Prayer." The prayer has the components of praise, adoration, exaltation, expression of our dependency on the will of God, petition, forgiveness, and protection from dangers and obstacles. It is a prayer that captured perfect expression of faith, hope, love, humility, and a total reliance on the will of God.

I also encourage Christian nurses to include practising mindfulness as a form of prayer, a reflective practice, and a way of life. The ability to ground oneself in the moment, to focus and fully immerse oneself in the present, and to be consciously aware of the meaning and the purpose of the events as they develop is a great skill. Mindfulness as a therapeutic practice could help prevent or reduce the frequency of compassion fatigue in nursing professional practice. Mindfulness is anchored in two important parts: self-regulation of attention and curious, non-judgmental orientation to present experience (Seigel, Germer & Olendzki, 2009). The Christian nurse needs to focus on the present while acknowledging and accepting the feelings, emotions, and physical bodily sensations they are experiencing in the present as a therapeutic technique to avoid being overwhelmed by what is happening at the moment. They should also do this to maintain a healthy outlook, and to adequately regulate their emotions.

The philosophy of mindfulness in nursing is grounded in the nurse's conscious awareness in the moment, so as to be aware of their thoughts and how these thoughts impact their experience. As human beings, we often find ourselves both consciously and unconscious drawn to unhelpful thinking. These unhelpful thoughts are mainly the products of our upbringing, nature, nurture, beliefs, values, and opinions, which inform and influence the lenses through which we view reality.

A practical example to demonstrate how worldviews, including the Christian worldview, could trigger unhelpful thinking is shown in Romans 3:23: "All have sinned and fallen short of the glory of God." Sometimes, Christians perseverate and fixate on the mistakes they made and the sins they committed, to the point that they experience extreme, irrational, and unhelpful guilt. To some extent, the feeling of guilt could lead one to healthy contrition, repentance, and the forgiveness of sins by God; however, extreme guilt could lead to cognitive distortions, which could translate to a psychopathology, especially in the areas of depression and anxiety disorders.

Sometimes, during the time of depression and anxiety, patients who have religious beliefs demonstrate unhelpful thinking, where they feel extreme guilt about the sins they committed, while possessing the image of God as an avenging God, who is taking note of their sins in order to punish them. These patients often perceive their physical or mental sickness as a punishment from God for the sins they committed in the past. The extreme guilt experienced by these patients could translate into doubt about whether God has actually totally forgiven them of their sins. It could also trigger their perception of any form of misfortune that comes their way as a punishment from God for the sins they committed. This way of thinking is unhelpful, to say the least.

I admonish the Christian nurse to recognize that Jesus died for our sins to set us free and to bring us the salvation from our sins. This assertion finds its vindication in (Romans 8: 1-3), as follows:

Therefore, there is now no condemnation for those who are in Christ Jesus because through Christ Jesus the law of the spirit who gives life has set you free from the law of sin and death. For what the law was powerless to do because it was weakened by the flesh, God did by sending his own Son in the likeness of sinful flesh to be a sin offering.

The practice of mindfulness by Christian nurses could help them to be consciously aware at all times, especially in those moments when they are maligned by the sense of guilt from the mistakes or the sins they committed, to focus on the prize paid for our sins by Christ. Since mindfulness is centred around being aware and being in the moment, it could help Christian nurses to be in control of their focus and attention; to control their wondering minds, and to remove their negative thoughts, which is often in a default mode that dominates and negatively impact their lives (Martin, 2015).

Instead of perseverating and fixating on the sins they committed and the mistakes they made, the Christian nurse should focus on the promises of Christ and the love and the forgiveness demonstrated by Jesus on the cross. They should be aware, through faith, that when God forgives us our sins, God also considers us as both righteous and sinless. My point is this: in the eyes of the God, we are sinless. Even when your colleagues see you as a failure, you are a winner in the eyes of God. They may write you off as being incompetent, but God sees you as a priceless masterpiece.

Grounded in the practice of mindfulness, I want the Christian nurse not to allow the guilt from the sins they committed or the mistakes they made to rob them of their inner peace and their confidence. Instead, I want them to focus on the following assertions well articulated in Osteen (2016):

> *God does not look on the outside; He looks at the heart. Even when we make mistakes, God doesn't write us off. He always gives us another chance. Why? Because God can see the eagle in the tree trunk. He can see the butterfly in the worms. He can see a champion in a failure. But it is up to us. The only way the transformation will begin is for you to believe that you are for-given, believe that there is mercy for every mistake, and believe you are who God says you are. (p. 64)*

I encourage the Christian nurse to meditate on the immensity and the depth of God's love for us, a love that is unconditional, a love that does not keep track of all the wrongs, mistakes, and sins we commit, a love that abounds even in the midst of our unfaithfulness. God is always faithful. God never gives up on us. God wants us to be happy. God wants us to be at peace. But we need to recognize these promises, believe in them, and claim them before they can come to fruition.

CHAPTER 10: Relying on God and Not on Humans in Nursing Practice

Trust in the Lord with all your heart; do not depend on your own understanding. Seek his will in all you do and he will show you which path to take.
—Proverbs 3: 5-6.

HUMAN BEINGS ARE social beings by nature. We love to socialize and associate with others. This necessary association underscores the simple fact that no one is an island. The natural yearning to start a relationship and interact with others often gives us sense of acceptance and belonging, especially with people that have similarities or common interests and occupations. Their acceptance seems to define us and become part of our identity. People tend to place their trust in human alliances and social networks at their workplace, believing that solidarity with a particular group of people at work will give them security and advance them to where they want to be. Relying and trusting on those they perceive as important in any workplace often comes with a false sense of hope, status, security, and importance. It sometimes reaches the point where they undermine and disregard others they judge as the commoners or the underachievers in the workplace.

Remember, there is nothing wrong with building healthy alliances and healthy social networks with the people you work with. Remember, there is nothing wrong with entering into a healthy relationship with people you work with. Remember that teamwork is an indispensable component of effective nursing.

It is a great feeling when we get along with our nursing colleagues and when they give us positive feedback on our performances at work and outside of work. Those compliments often make us feel better, while positively impacting our confidence and reaffirming our sense of belonging with our work community. It is important to have basic trust in the people who you work with. This basic trust is necessary for competent teamwork.

It is a fundamentally flawed idea to rely on people from your workplace as the source of your confidence and sense of self. It is both unhealthy and dangerous to rely on the emotional validation, affirmation, and acceptance of people you work with for your happiness and fulfilment. Often, people who are desperate for acceptance or to associate with those they perceive as powerful in nursing for security have issues with their own self esteem, lack of self-confidence, and feelings of incompetence. Nursing is a career where over eighty percent of nurses belong to a specific gender, and there is nothing wrong with that. Bullying and other workplace violence in nursing are strongly documented, and nurses' bullying could involve verbal aggression and gossip. One thing I know, based on my extensive nursing experience, is that there is a lot of talk among nurses. There are a lot of opinions and feedback, both constructive and destructive. In nursing, you will have both champions and detractors. It is therefore wrong to rely on people's comments, judgments, and acceptance for your happiness. It is a great knowledge and wisdom to rely on God at all times and to seek God's approval and acceptance instead. In a pragmatic sense, God never fails. God never lies to us. God never slanders us, and He will not make fun of us or celebrate our weaknesses, for it is not in the nature of God to do those things. Instead, God understands our pain and wants us to come to Him for rest and peace from our problems.

I want Christian nurses to understand that they will have both supporters and challengers among colleagues and patients in nursing. I want Christian nurses to be comfortable with this indispensable reality of the presence of detractors in nursing workplaces, which are often complex and demanding. It is very easy to get along with colleagues and patients who say good things about you, and it could be devastating for some nurses when they are confronted by colleagues who are their antagonists. I want Christian nurses to perceive their antagonists at work as their greatest helpers and to perceive the people that wrestle with them as making them strong, as asserted by Edmund Burke.

In your experience of destructive feedback from a colleague who is your detractor and antagonist, do not be moved, and do not lose your professional behaviour. Instead, keep calm and remember the following assertions from Osteen (2016):

> *People may not approve you. Don't worry about it. God approves you.*
>
> *People didn't call you. People don't determine your destiny. People can't stop God's plan in your life. God called you. God equipped you.*
>
> *God anointed you. When you come to the end of your life, you don't have to answer to people. You will answer to Almighty God. (p. 150)*

The Christian nurse should understand that God is the source of happiness and every blessing. God never fails, but sometimes, human beings can fail us. Friends can sometimes disappoint us. Friends can let us down, especially when the going gets tough. The story of the passion and death of Jesus in the Bible showed that the apostle Peter, who was very close to Jesus and who promised to stand by Jesus at all times, including at the darkest moments, denied Jesus three times when Jesus needed him the most. Human beings are not perfect beings, and they can let you down. A good friend can sometimes disappoint you, especially during difficult times.

Friends, it is better to rely on God than to rely on humans. The Bible echoed in several instances the need to rely and trust God instead of relying on humans. That God is a perfect God, a faithful God, an all-powerful God, an all-knowing God, and an all-loving God are statements of faith, which we believe to be true and have experienced in our lives in one way or the other. When you rely on God and trust in God at all times and in all circumstances, the God of miracles will begin to do the impossible in your life. It does not imply that the Christian nurse who relied on God will not go through difficult times every now and then. It is utopic to believe that, for such is a false hope. Rather, my point is that the God of miracles who turned water into wine in Galilee is bigger than any trouble or any obstacle that you may experience.

Relying on, and trusting in God comes with a lot of benefits. First, you will experience the lasting peace that comes from trusting in God. As the book of Isaiah echoed: "You keep him in perfect peace whose mind is stayed on you, because he trusts in you (Isaiah 26: 3-4). Second, when we trust in God, we receive abundant blessing from God, as evidenced in the book of Psalm: "Blessed is the one who trusts in the Lord" (34:8). Third, the Lord will quickly come to your aid and offer His continual protection and shield as the Psalmist declared: "And the Lord shall help them, deliver them: he shall deliver them from the wicked and save them, because they trust in him" (Psalm 37:40). Fourth, when you trust in the Lord, God will take care of your needs and make you fruitful and prosperous: "Blessed is the one who trusts in the Lord, whose confidence is in him. They will be like a tree planted by the water that sends out its roots by the stream. It does not fear when heat comes; its leaves are always green" (Jeremiah 17:7-8).

In the book of Psalms, the psalmist echoed that "it is better to take refuge in the Lord than to trust in princes" (Psalm 118:9). Moreover, "do not put your confidence in powerful people; there is no help for you there" (Psalm 146:3). The book of Psalms underscored the frailty of humans and the imperfection evidenced in human nature, which often translates to disappointments and betrayals, making it unwise to fully trust and rely on human beings and wise to trust and rely on God, who never fails or changes. Evident in the book of Hebrews 13:8 is the assertion that "Jesus Christ is the same yesterday, today and forever." God never changes. Indeed, "the steadfast love of the Lord never ceases; his mercies never come to an end; they are new every morning; great is your faithfulness" (Lamentations 3:22-23). There are several instances in the Bible where the need to trust and rely on God alone as opposed to human beings were highlighted.

Friends, if you rely on, and trust in God, He will take you to the place you need to be and lead you to your destiny, or to the position where you aspire to be in your nursing profession. I encourage every Christian nurse to dream big dreams, to strive for excellence in practice, and to do all things within their power to continue to present themselves as competent nurses who are fully prepared to effectively care for their patients. I encourage Christian nurses to form the habit of continuously enhancing their knowledge and continuing their effort for competence in practice. If you do what is in your power to become the best, God will open doors that human beings will never open for you. God will lift you and set you up where you need to be in life at the right time.

Lastly, I encourage Christian nurses not to waste their time in kowtowing to the whims of people with power in their workplace or to engage in sycophantic behaviour, for that is simply a demonstration of superficiality. Rather, be genuine and authentic to everyone. I encourage Christian nurses to be cosmopolitan in their workplace, where they show respect and love for everyone, and where they demonstrate open-mindedness in appreciating the differences that each person brings, and to understand that those differences do not need to be fully resolved for them to get along with others (Appiah, 2006). I encourage Christian nurses to define themselves as authentic and genuine at work, to maintain emotional stability and competence in their nursing practice, and to make their behaviour predictable to others. Above all, I encourage Christian nurses to ground their nursing practice in knowledge and in prayer, to trust in God, and to rely on God alone at all times, and in all circumstances, with the knowledge that "strong lions suffer want and go hungry, but those who trust in the Lord will lack no blessings" (Psalm 34:10). Friends, we need to trust in God at all times and continue to ask God to increase our faith (Luke 17:5).

CHAPTER 11: Nursing Through the Lens of a Christian Worldview

Many people have the Bible in their heads, or in their pockets; but we need to get it down into our hearts.
—D.L. Moody.

SOCIAL SCIENTISTS OFTEN contend that human beings are products of nature and nurture to buttress how the environment, including the people we interact and relate with, especially our families, play in the formation of our identity and worldview. As we relate and interact with one another, we realize the obvious reality of the existence of differences in worldviews and our perceptions of reality. We encounter differences of opinions, differences in beliefs and assumptions, differences in the way we understand and interpret the world around us, differences in what we perceive as values, differences on how we ascribe meaning to realities, and differences in how we determine what is meaningful. At the core of our human interactions and relationships is the reality of differences in worldviews.

Elaborating on the existence and beauty of different worldviews, opinions, values, and belief systems held by the people we encounter, Appiah (2006) asserted that "people are different, and there is much to learn from our differences. Because there are so many human possibilities worth exploring, we neither expect nor desire everyone or every society should converge on a single mode of life" (p.xv). The different beliefs, cultural values, and religious values we possess inform and influence the worldview we possess, which is the lens through which we view reality.

What, then, is worldview? Worldview is the conglomeration of assumptions or beliefs we have about the world and the events we experience, which affect how we think and live. The core values, ideas, and beliefs that individuals hold inform and influence their thoughts and behaviours (Cosgrove, 2006). A person who has strong faith in God and the Bible as the word of God, for example, will try to reflect their biblical beliefs in their actions and their relationship with others. The values, assumptions, and cultural and family beliefs consciously or unconsciously influence the way we think and do things; sometimes, they determine what we think and inform the lenses through which we see realities. Our worldviews affect the way we see things and help us to have a clearer perception of things, just like the glasses help some people to have a clear view of things (Cosgrove, 2006). Indeed, worldview is like a puzzle box top picture or image. The pieces of pictures are like life experiences and the knowledge we have about things and how things should be. With this puzzle box image, which serves as a guide/framework, one will be able to put the pieces of scattered pictures together into a meaningful image. That's what worldview does to human beings (Cosgrove, 2006).

A comprehensive and all-inclusive understanding of worldview was articulated by Sire (2009) as:

> *A commitment, a fundamental orientation of the heart that can be expressed as a story or in a set of presuppositions (assumptions which may be true, partially true or entirely false) that we hold (consciously or subconsciously, consistently or inconsistently) about the basic constitution of reality, and that provides the foundation on which we live and move and have our being. (p. 20)*

It is also important to point out that sometimes, our worldviews are not always based on fact or truth. Our worldviews can be fragmented and inconsistent. Since human experience is both lived and shared, we impact people with whom we come in contact, and we ourselves are also impacted by the people we interact and relate with. In the process of our interaction and relationship with one another, we are bound to see people who possess and act on a belief system, and who hold worldviews, that are not based on truth. People have committed different atrocities, and we have experienced violent terrorist acts for example, due to some people possessing worldviews that are not factual and that are inhuman. Cosgrove (2006) asserted that "we also must help people improve upon their worldviews when their beliefs have inconsistencies or when their assumptions are not in agreement with good information" (p. 28).

I consider myself a cosmopolitan. By that, I mean that I tolerate, accept, and respect differences of worldviews, and I believe that we have responsibility to one another, which includes helping to improve each other's worldview and belief system, when they are not grounded on fact and on truth in the context of today. Sometimes, we need to engage in thoughtful deliberation and discussion with people to understand the belief system behind what they do. We must enter those deliberations with open minds and with the acceptance that sometimes those different worldviews, especially the atrocious ones that negatively infringe on other people's lives and people's rights, may not be a settled opinion. I encourage Christian nurses to take a cosmopolitan stance in their workplace and be driven by a cosmopolitan curiosity when relating and interacting with others. I encourage them to take a non-judgmental stance that opens the door for understanding different worldviews without sacrificing their core values and Christian worldviews.

Characteristics of Worldview

There are different characteristics of worldview. First, worldview is a commitment, and the essence of the worldview we possess lies at the very core of human persons—the heart (Sire, 2009). Our beliefs and assumptions, which are important to us, are held dearly in our heart and soul, and we are committed to those religious and cultural beliefs, assumptions, and values, for they are the primary motivators of what we do and how we behave.

Second, worldview is demonstrated and communicated in the form of a story (Sire, 2009). Although worldview is not a story in a strict sense, it is expressed as a narrative. Each of us has a story and a narrative that inform and influence how we see the world. This story is a conglomeration of all the knowledge we receive from our family, our experiences, and formal and informal education. For Christians, for example, the story of the Fall and the story of the suffering and death of Jesus are of great importance. All these narratives, which we hold so dearly in our heart, inform and influence how we make sense of our reality.

Third, worldview may or not be based on truth. The assumptions and beliefs we possess may be based on right information and on truth. It can be partially true or completely false (Sire, 2009). Sometimes, the assumption and beliefs we hold about something are simply part of the story of our lives, and we don't really have a full understanding of the reason why we believe or hold firmly to a particular value, but we know that it is how everyone around us has behaved, and as such, it becomes central to how we think and behave. It is a fact that sometimes, appearance differs from reality, and as such, we need to approach people with open mind, especially when we deliberate and negotiate on the meaning of beliefs and assumptions.

Fourth, Worldview is both fundamental and foundational to our lives (Sire, 2009). The worldviews we hold are the primary determinant of how we think and the actions we take. Worldview is foundational to making meaning of the world around us. It is embedded in the essence of who we are, in the core of our heart. It is so automatic and subconscious in our thought and behaviour that we often need scrupulous examination and rigorous reflection to be consciously aware of them, including the potential bias that comes with them. It becomes necessary to engage in reflective practice, to be able to identify the bias we subconsciously hold the reality around us, especially in our relationship with people and our decision-making process, making sure that we align our thoughts and actions on truth and right information. What, then, is a Biblical or Christian worldview?

Christian Worldview

Our worldviews have significant impact on how we feel and what we do, especially in times of difficulty, illness, and pain. During unpleasant times, for example, Christians turn to God for help and comfort. Also, during a good time, such as the birth of a child, Christians turn to God for thanksgiving and to ask for God's blessings on the newborn. In the worldview they possess, that a child is a gift from God, and that God is the source and the giver of life. Christian worldview is therefore central to how Christians live, think, and behave.

The important aspect of Christian worldview is grounded in its attempt to give all inclusive and comprehensive understanding of the reality that is anchored in the word of God and give meaning and interpretation to the events in the universe (Naugle, 2002). A Christian worldview, or rather a biblical worldview, is the expression of what the human grasps of the underlying revelations in Scripture. It is an effort by human beings, who are finite and limited, to understand what God has revealed in the Scripture within human limitations (Hiebert, 2008).

To have a full understanding of the Bible requires relentless effort to grasp the background, the themes, and its underlying central message, the person of Christ. It is a fundamental flaw to presume that we have full understanding of the biblical worldview (Hiebert, 2008). The central themes that undergird the Christian worldview are the belief that God is the creator of the universe, that human beings were created by God, that God revealed Himself in creatures, that God is love, that human knowledge is finite, and that God is infinite, to mention but a few (Hiebert, 2008). The basic concept of God in biblical or Christian worldview is that God is infinite; God is personal (and triune as well); God is transcendent; God is omniscience; God is sovereign; and God is good (Sire, 2009).

A practising Christian who is also a nurse should be influenced by their Christian worldview, directly or indirectly, consciously or unconsciously, in their care of the patients. The Christian nurse's understanding and belief in the existence of God, who is immanent, all-loving, all-caring, and who has commissioned Christians to spread the message of love by loving their neighbours as themselves, should inform and influence the Christian nurses' lenses of nursing practice.

Central to Christian worldview and belief is the idea that God is the giver of life, that life is sacred, and that human beings are the custodians of their lives. As such, to be a good custodian and steward who is created in the image and likeness of God, human beings are therefore expected to do all things necessary, reasonable, and ethical to preserve themselves in being, which includes taking good care of their health.

The Christian nurse should not lose sight of the fact that it is necessary to use an empirical worldview as well in their nursing practice, since it also underscores and perceives health in holistic context, and it affirms the idea of healing of the whole person—physically, emotionally, mentally, and spiritually—as opposed to the absence of physical illness only.

I assert that the idea of holistic nursing care that accounts for the individual's mental health, physical health, emotional health and spiritual needs, is consistent and aligns with the Christian worldview of healing and caring for the whole person, as evidenced in the work and the ministry of Jesus. There are several instances and narratives in the Scriptures, especially in the New Testament, that demonstrated the healing actions of Jesus transcending the healing of a physical illness to the healing of the whole person.

Evident in the synoptic gospel is Jesus's commitment to the healing of the whole person and restoring health to people in holistic context. The human person is composed of body organs and body parts that are interdependent and interconnected. Whenever someone is sick, for example, that sickness impacts the whole person's mind, emotion, and spirituality as well. For human beings to function effectively at their optimal level, the organs and all the parts of the body must be reasonably functioning efficiently.

Sickness affects the whole person. In the Christian worldview, sin also impacts the whole person. More importantly, in the Christian worldview, we understand that through the blood Jesus shed on the cross, Christians are forever liberated and saved from the power of sin and death. As such, there is always mercy, love, and forgiveness anytime we reach out to God.

From this point of view, therefore, it is not uncommon or out of context to see Jesus' actions during the time of His ministry as being focused on healing the whole person. The Christian nurse should be consciously aware that the idea of healing the whole person, evident in health/empirical world-view, is not radically distant and distinct from the Christian worldview's understanding of healing of the whole person, as demonstrated by Jesus during His work and ministry, despite the differences in the method and in the manner of their therapeutic interventions.

Evident in the gospel of Mark, Chapter 2, is the story of Jesus healing a paralyzed man by first saying to him, "your sins are forgiven" before healing the paralyzed man's physical sickness by telling him to "get up, take your mat and walk." These assertions from Jesus demonstrate and underscore the fact that Jesus perceives health and wellness in a holistic context, and Jesus took care of the emotional and spiritual needs of the sick by forgiving the sins the paralyzed man committed.

Jesus never lost sight of the people's emotional needs during His work and ministry on earth. When He noticed that they were tired and suffering from fatigue due to their work, Jesus admonished his disciples to, "come with me by yourselves to a quiet place and get some rest" (Mark 6:31).

Jesus also cared for the social needs of the people. This assertion is evident in several instances in the bible, especially in the stories of Jesus' healings and miracles. In Luke, Chapter 17, Jesus healed ten men who had leprosy. The men stood at a distance because they were excommunicated from the community due to their sickness, and they were not allowed to come close to people. The ten men who were suffering from leprosy cried out and shouted from a distance, "Jesus, master, have pity on us" (Luke 17: 13). People suffering from leprosy were excommunicated from the rest of the community, and they were required to shout, "unclean" when they encounter people on their way. Jesus healed the ten men from their leprosy, and He restored them back to the community from which they were severed, feeling abandoned with lack of sense of belonging and connectedness.

These actions and practical examples of Jesus are part of the narratives, stories, assumptions, and beliefs that translate to a Christian worldview, from which the Christian nurse operates. These biblical worldviews undergird Christian nurses' understanding of caring, health, and recovery from sickness. It is a popular Christian belief that God is present everywhere, including in the workplace and our activities of daily living. The Christian nurse can touch the lives of people in the workplace and extend the presence of God to their patients and colleagues.

Jesus was often shown in the Bible to be moved with compassion, and He was filled with empathy, especially for the sick, the weak, the poor, and the oppressed. Genuine empathy and compassion are evident in the life and work of Jesus, are also essential component of Christian worldview, and they should guide and influence the Christian nurse's patient care. They should also become the essence of who they are and the foundation on which they build their nursing practice.

Nursing within a Christian worldview is not in sharp contrast with the health science paradigm or the health science worldview, especially regarding the necessity and relevancy of the healing of the whole person. Although, there may be some differences on the implications and approaches to health and wellness by both the scientific worldview and Christian worldview, the goal is still the same.

Elaborating on the complementarity of the Christian worldview with empirical or scientific worldview, Shelly and Miller (2006) asserted that "Christian worldview affirms good empirical science and appropriate use of technology. They are gifts from God to be used for the benefit of creation" (p. 52). Evidenced in creationism, or the story of creation in the biblical context (Genesis 1:28), is the fact that God created the world and commanded humans to "increase and multiply; to fill the earth, and to subdue it." The emphasis here is on the world "subdue," and in our context, this extends to include the invention and use of appropriate technology and scientific paradigm that is anchored in the ethical principles of beneficence and non-maleficence, as the extension of God's commission to human beings.

Our worldviews inform our perception of events, our decision and judgment of situations in our lives, and our sensemaking of reality. They also serve as the bedrock or the foundation of our nursing practice. The Christian worldview is anchored in the truth revealed in the Bible. Christian nurses, therefore, should be influenced by their Christian worldview, together with their health and nursing science worldview, in their care of the patients.

Christian nurses often value and aspire towards nursing model that is consistent with their values and belief, and not toward the models that are in sharp contrast with their beliefs and Christian worldview. Elaborating on this idea, Eckerd (2018) asserted:

Christian nurses need models upon which they can align their practice—models based on the agape love characteristics of Christ. Useful not only in nursing but also in life, the goal of such a model is to allow the spirit of God to dominate situations and reflect the heart and character of Christ. (p. 2)

Eckerd (2018) located such a model in Agape model, which is a nursing practice that is influenced by the actions and behaviours of Jesus, through the inspiration of the Holy Spirit, and evidenced and witnessed in the life of the nurse. The Agape model for nursing practice is therefore the manifestation of the character which is Agape love through the nurse's practice, a genuine and unconditional love that Jesus has shown to all of us—sinners, strangers, and unbelievers.

The Christian nurse who practises with the theology and the mindset of Agape love is the one who is both human and humane, who perceives every patient as a reflection of the image of the invisible God, who practises with unconditional love to all, including patients and colleagues with different values and worldviews, and who understands the sacredness of human life.

The Christian nurse, who uses the Christian worldview as a guide for nursing practice, should be able to embrace the Agape model because it is better aligned with their values and beliefs. The Christian nurse should perceive nursing practice as a call or a vocation to care for the sick and the wounded within the context of nursing professional practice, as opposed to merely having a nursing job, per se.

Eckerd (2018) underscored four basic assumptions or constructs that accurately captured the meaning and the context of Agape love, using the acronym as follows: "A—Accept

Christ as saviour, G—Grow spiritually and professionally, A—Anticipate Holy Spirit intervention, P—Prayer and spiritual gifts, E—Embrace the fruit of the Spirit" (p. 48). In other words, Christian nurses who practise with Agape model, grounded in a Christian worldview, should be authentic believers in Christ, who aspire to grow both professionally and personally through prayer and spiritual gifts. They are able to assess the needs of the patients entrusted to their care while relying on their nursing knowledge and the inspiration from the Holy Spirit, and they reflect on the gifts of the spirits, such as love, joy, peace, patience, kindness, goodness, faithfulness, gentleness and self-control (Galatians 5), while caring for their patients.

The philosophy and theology of the Agape love model evident in the biblical worldview, as seen in the characters and qualities of Jesus, aligns with professional nursing, as it was envisioned by Florence Nightingale. The analysis of the content, context, and meaning of Agape love highlights the need for the Christian nurse who uses the model to aspire to grow in empirical ways of knowing in nursing practice and to advance in spirituality. Also, the nurse needs to continue to care for patients in holistic contexts.

If the Christian nurse is fully committed to the assumptions that undergird the concept of Agape love, the nurse could be better equipped to practise competently. The nurse who is committed to the constructs of Agape love model could be adorned with the necessary qualities, such as love, compassion, empathy, and knowledge, to mention but a few, which Jesus Christ demonstrated in caring for the sick and the wounded, the poor and the oppressed. These qualities

Lawrence Onwuegbuchunam, Ph.D., RN.

demonstrated by Jesus during His life and ministry are both necessary and relevant for effective nursing practice in our society today.

So, What Then? Putting it Together. Thinking it Through.

Nursing is firmly rooted in Christian tradition and religious principles. The role of Roman Catholic nuns in the advancement of nursing stands as a pragmatic and concrete justification and vindication of the underlying religious significance of nursing, at least, from historical perspective. The idea of caring for the sick and rendering service to the poor, the wounded, and the stranger, is not distant and distinct from what Christians are called to do, and it is not an elusive concept within the Christian worldview. Currently, nursing is a regulated profession, and as such, for the Christian nurse, and within the Christian worldview, nursing could be understood and perceived both as a call or vocation from God and a profession (career).

Christian values and qualities, such as compassion, empathy, caring, service, commitment, love, and knowledge, to mention but a few, are fundamental and foundational to professional nursing, and they are central to the understanding of the meaning and the context of competent and effective nursing. As nursing practice continues to evolve and expand, more attention seems to be given to the scientific and empirical worldview in a quest for recognition and acceptance as a professional practice, while detaching any religious significance to the meaning of the care and service that nurses provide. I admonish the Christian nurse to see nursing as a calling from God and as a profession, for both concepts are not mutually exclusive.

Spirituality is an essential and central component of humans. The search for meaning, purpose, belonging, and acceptance, is central to human beings in general, and it is particularly important to majority of the patients that nurses work with, especially during patients' illness experiences and recovery journey. The spiritual component of nursing assessments and interventions in a holistic context cannot be denied. The notion of holistic nursing assessments and interventions can never be complete without the inclusion of the nurse's spiritual assessment of patient's needs and spiritual intervention, including sending referrals to the facility's chaplain, provision of relevant community resources, and making connections with religious community agencies.

Nursing is among the most respected careers due to the essential work that nurses do. Also, most of the people that came to nursing simply want to give their best, sincerely care for patients entrusted to their care, and positively impact and contribute to patients' recovery and well-being. They do so with a deep sense of satisfaction and fulfilment at the end of the day, knowing that they made a difference in peoples' lives and that they made an honest living.

It is also a statement of fact, grounded in nursing literature, that some nurses sometimes eat their young and one another in their work environment. The reality of aggression, especially verbal and passive aggression in nursing professional practice, cannot be denied. The presence of hostility, bullying, gossiping, backstabbing, unfair patient assignment, and destructive criticisms that could destroy the morale of colleagues, to mention but a few, have been experienced by some nurses in their workplace.

The Christian nurse is not immune from experiencing aggression and hostility at work. The Christian nurse needs to make conscious effort, on a daily basis, not to be part of the perpetrators of workplace aggression and hostility. Rather, they must strive to treat both patients and professional colleagues with love, because love is foundational to what it means to be a Christian. Also, the Christian nurse should take the necessary steps and explore the established avenues for dealing with any form of aggression and harassment in their workplace.

The Christian should be consciously aware of the fact that they have ethical, moral, and professional responsibilities to speak up when they see unsafe nursing care, including ethical and moral misconduct, despite the challenges and obstacles, both internal and external obstacles that come with speaking up or whistleblowing. Moral courage is a quality that every Christian nurse should possess.

The Christian nurse has an obligation to demonstrate a fitness to practise. This fitness to practise extends to include making sure that they come to work fully prepared: mentally, physically, emotionally, and spiritually, to function at their optimal level, and to minimize or eradicate the chances of error, especially medication error. When the Christian nurse has taken all the due diligence to practise safely, and errors occur due to human nature, they should not be despaired—or worse still, they should not try to cover up the error due to potential repercussions or consequences of medication error.

Rather, the Christian nurse should always remember that God is closer to his people during difficult and trying times. They should remember to trust God and to follow the steps established by their work facilities for handling adverse incidents, especially medication errors. The Christian nurse should strive to avoid making mistakes at work because of the proximity of those errors to peoples' lives, while being consciously aware of the sacredness of human lives. But in the event of human error, they should accept their mistakes and see the mistake as an opportunity for learning and for professional growth.

While caring for the patients, the Christian nurse should perceive therapeutic communication with patients as an opportunity to actively listen to the patient and immerse themselves into their stories to fully understand their needs, and what is pertinent to them. This will allow them to plan intervention that is relevant, specific to patients' needs, and effective. The Christian nurse should not be afraid to assess the spiritual needs of the patients. And, if patients proactively start the discussion on the belief in the existence of God and note submission to the will of God as one of their coping mechanisms, the Christian nurse should not shy away from exploring that topic about the relevancy of God in their illness journey, while making sure that they are not affirming delusions of religious type, and that they are not giving patients false hope. In other words, the Christian nurse has to be consciously aware of both the constructive and the destructive impacts of religious beliefs or spirituality in illness recovery well documented in literature.

The role of the nurse is critical. It is a role that has direct impact on the lives of the patients. Due to the nature of the work that nurses do, it is ethically, professionally, and morally imperative that Christian nurses value and embrace punctuality in their practice and understand that the duty of care is the responsibility they owe to their patients. Nurses work collaboratively with other professionals, and teamwork is an indispensable aspect or component of effective nursing care. It is an understatement to say that a Christian nurse should be a good and a reliable team player. Indeed, Christian nurses should be leaders and major contributors to effective and efficient teamwork that facilitate and promote competent nursing care, and should be aware that tardiness is grievously frowned upon in nursing practice.

While rigorously investing and immersing themselves in the care of their patients, Christian nurses should not forget their need for self-care if they wish to avoid the issue of burnout in their nursing practice. Nurses often work in an environment where trauma, pain, and death are present. The workplace becomes even more challenging to nurses in general, and to the Christian nurse in particular, in our context, if the culture of the workplace is oppressive and unsupportive of the needs of patients and staff. The effect of toxic workplace could translate to the burnout of nurses.

The nurse who does self-care, and who is consciously aware of their limits, energy level, strengths, and weaknesses, and who understands when to take a break to rejuvenate or reinvigorate their energy level through relaxation techniques, is doing something good to themselves, which could also translate to being a good steward to the patients. The

Christian nurse should therefore strive to create a balance and maintain hemostasis in their physical, mental, emotional and spiritual wellbeing. The Christian nurse's self-knowledge and self-awareness could help them develop strategies and healthy coping skills that are relevant, necessary, reasonable, and specific to their self-care needs.

In line with the concept of self-care, Christian nurses need to ground their nursing practice in prayer. They need to make prayer the foundation of their nursing practice while being consciously aware of the St. Augustine's assertion that human souls are restless until they rest in the God. Christian nurses should be aware that there are many instances in the Bible that underscore the idea of prayer, and surrendering to God, as a way to find rest, security, and peace of mind and body. Indeed, nursing can be both stressful and demanding, although it is rewarding as well. It is therefore both necessary and compulsory that Christian nurses anchor themselves in God, together with their nursing practice, as a perfect strategy to reduce stress and enjoy the blessing, the satisfaction, and the fulfilment that come with rendering service and caring for the sick, as promised in the Bible.

Friends, it is better to trust in God, and to rely on God, than to put your hope and trust in human beings. One with God is majority. Nursing is both an independent and collaborative practice, where it is necessary to have basic trust with the nursing team to give competent care to the patients. Basic trust is also necessary for establishing and building healthy workplace alliances. But it is a fundamentally flawed idea to rely on people as sources of confidence or self-worth. Remember that a friend today could be your enemy tomorrow.

God is your best friend. God never changes. God never fails. I cannot overemphasize this fact.

Friends, it is important to continue to evaluate the worldview you possess, including your Christian worldview, making sure that the ideas and beliefs you possess are grounded on truth and are aligned with right information. While holding on to your Christian worldview, do not lose sight of making sure that they are aligned with the nursing/health worldview and the standard set by the regulatory body in your jurisdiction for competent nursing practice. Allow both worldviews to inform and influence the lens of your nursing practice. Remember that nursing is a regulated profession.

May the love of God and your neighbour, which is the summary of the Law and the Prophets, as written in the Bible, be the foundation of your nursing practice. Remember that biblical truth is often context-specific. Remember that the Bible was written over many years ago, but the message, the truth, and the teaching of the Bible are still relevant and necessary as a guide to our lives today. Remember that the Bible needs to be interpreted and applied in the context of today.

Remember that the same Bible that said: "many are the trials of the just, but from them all the Lord will rescue them (Psalm 34:19), also said in second Corinthians Chapter 12, 8-9, "three times I plead the Lord to take away (this torn) from me. But he said to me, my grace is sufficient for you, for my power is made perfect in weakness." If we always remember that God loves us unconditionally, that God is all-knowing and all-caring, we will be able to submit to God, whatever comes our way, and still be at peace with the outcome of whatever comes our way in our nursing practice and our lives in general.

This is my contribution, and my admonitions to nurses who are practising Christians, on the issues in nursing professional practice, through the lens of a Christian worldview. This is my contribution toward the improvement and the mitigation of the issues evident in nursing professional practice from empirical and pragmatic perspectives, through the lens of a Christian worldview.

REFERENCES

Augustine of Hippo (2015). *Confessions*. Xist Publishing Company.

Appiah, K.W. (2006). *Cosmopolitanism: Ethics in a world of strangers*. W.W Norton & Company Press.

Ashurst, A. (2009). The consequences of whistleblowing. *Nursing & Residential Care, 11*(6), p.274.

Baesler, E.J. (2003). *Theoretical exploration and empirical investigation of communication and prayer*. Edwin Mellen Press.

Ball, E. (2013). Evolution of contemporary nursing. In Brooker, C. & Waugh, A. (Ed). *Foundations of nursing practice* (2nd ed., pp.33-60). Elsevier.

Bartholomew, K. (2006*). Ending hostility in nursing: Why nurses eat their young and each other*. Marblehead, MA: HCPro.

Bradshaw, A. (2002). *The nurse apprentice 1860-1977*. Aldershot, England: Ashgate.

Canadian Nurses Association (CNA). (1999). I see am silent. I see and I speak out: The dilemma of whistleblowing. *Ethics in Practice*. Retrieved from https://www.cna-aiic.ca/en.

Carter, M. (2014). Vocation and altruism in nursing: The habits of practice. *Nursing Ethics, 21*(6), 695-701. Doi:10.1177/0969733013516159.

Cheragi, M.A., Manoocheri, H., Mohammadnejad, E. & Ehsani, S. (2013). Types and causes of medication errors from nurse's viewpoint. *Iran Journal of Nurse Midwifery Res.* *18*(3). 228-231.

Canadian Nurses Association (CNA). (2002). *Nursing leadership*. Retrieved from https://www.cna-aiic.ca/en.

Cosgrove, M. (2006). *Foundations of Christian thought: Faith, learning and Christian worldview*. Kregel Publishers.

Dein, S., Cook, C., Powell, A., & Eagger, S. (2010) Religion, spirituality and mental health. *The Psychiatrist, 34*, (7), pp. 63-64. doi:10.1192/pb.109.025924.

Dewey, J. (1933). *How we think: A restatement of the relation of reflective thinking to the educative process*. D.C. Heath and Company.

Eckerd, N. (2018). A nursing practice model based on Christ: The Agape model. *Journal of Christian Nursing.* 35(2), p. 124-130.

Fallot, R.D. (2001). Spirituality and religion in psychiatric rehabilitation and recovery from illness. *International Review of Psychiatry, 13*, 110-116.

Greenleaf, R. K. (1991). *Servant leadership: A journey into the nature of legitimate power and greatness*. Paulist Press.

Helmstadter, C. & Godden, J. (2013). *Nursing before Nightingale, 1815-1899*. Ashgate Publishing.

Hiebert, P.G. (2008). Transforming worldviews: An anthropological understanding of how people change. Baker Academic.

Houston, C.J. (2006). *Professional issues in nursing: Challenges and opportunities*. Lippincott Williams & Wilkins.

Kao, L. (2001). Students corner. Nurses and whistleblowing: Is it worth it? *Maryland Nurse, 2*(3), 7-8.

Keatings, M., & Smith, O. (2000). *Ethical and legal issues in Canadian nursing* (2nd ed). Elsevier.

Kerr, J. R., & MacPhal, J. (1991). *Canadian nursing: Issues and perspectives*. Mosby-Year Books.

Kidder, R. M. (2003). *Moral courage*. Harper Collins.

Martin, P. (2015). *Coping and thriving in nursing: An essential guide to practice*. SAGE Journals.

Maslach, C. & Leiter, M.P. (2005). Reversing burnout: *How to rekindle your passion for work*. Retrieved from: researchgate.net.

Miller, L. (2013). Legal issues and risk management: what you should know before you "blow": Nurses and whistle-blowing in healthcare. *The Journal of Perinatal & Neonatal Nursing. 27*(3), 201-202.

Naugle, D.K. (2002). *Worldview: The history of a concept*. Eerdmans Publishing.

Northouse, P. G. (2013). *Leadership: Theory and practice* (6th ed.). Sage O' Brien, M.E. (2011). *Spirituality in nursing: Standing on holy ground (4th ed.)*. Jones & Bartlett.

O'Brien, M. E. (2011). *Servant leadership in nursing: Spirituality and practice in contemporary health care*. Jones and Bartlett.

Onwuegbuchunam, L. (2020). *Servant leadership and moral courage in Canadian nursing*. Friesen Press.

Osteen, J. (2016). *Think better live better: A victorious life beings in your mind*. Faith Words.

Petterson, E.F. (1998). The philosophy and physics of holistic care: Spiritual healing as a workable interpretation. *Journal of Advanced Nursing, 27*, 287-293.

Pohl, C.D. (1999). *Making room: Recovering spirituality as a Christian tradition*. Eerdmans.

Roach, M.S. (2002) *Caring, the human mode of being: A blueprint for the health professions*. CHA Press.

Rosdahl, C.B. & Kowalski, M.T. (2008). *Textbook of basic nursing (9th ed.).* Lippincott William & Wilkens.

Ross, C. (1994). Spiritual aspect of nursing. *Journal of Advance Nursing, 19,* 439-447.

Rousseau, P. (2000). The art of oncology: When the tumour is not the target. Death denial. *Journal of Clinical Oncology,* 18, 3998-3999.

Roy, C. (1984). *Introduction to nursing: An adaptation model.* Prentice Hall.

Shelley, J.A. & Miller, A.B. (2006). *Called to care: A Christian worldview for nursing.* InterVarsity Press.

Siegel, R.D., Germer, C.K. & Olendzki, A. (2009). Mindfulness: What is it? Where did it come From? In F. Didonna (Ed.), *General handbook of mindfulness* (pp.17-35). Springer.

Sire, J.W. (2009). *The universe next door: A basic worldview catalog (5th ed.).* IVP Academic.

Spears, L. (2010). Character and servant leadership: Ten characteristics of effective caring leaders. *Journal of Virtues & Leadership, 1,* 25-30. Retrieved from https://www.regent.edu/acad/global/publications/jvl/vol1_iss1/Spears_Final.pdf.

Stumpf, E.S. & Fieser, J. (2008). *Philosophy: History and problems (7th ed.).* McGraw Hill.

Turton, D.W. & Francis, L.J. (2007). The relationship between attitude toward prayer and Professional burnout among Anglican parochial clergy in England: Are praying Clergy healthier clergy? *Religion and Culture, 10*(1), 61-74.

Water, T., Ramussen, S., Neufield, M., Gerrald, D., & Ford, K. (2017). Nursing's duty of care: From legal obligation to moral commitment. *Nursing Praxis in New Zealand. 33*(3), pp. 7-20.

9 781039 108776